BRAIN RESCUE

A 90 Day Blueprint to Reclaim Your Memory After a Brain Injury or Concussion

START YOUR RECOVERY JOURNEY TODAY!

DR. BRODY MILLER, PHD

PRAISE FOR DR. BRODY & BRAIN RESCUE

"Brain Rescue is a life-changing guide for anyone recovering from brain trauma. Packed with cutting-edge neuroscience, it's a beacon of hope that empowers readers to reclaim their health and their future."

- **John Assaraf,** CEO of Neurogym and 2x NY Times Bestselling Author

"There are no coincidences in life... and when I met Dr. Brody Miller, I found him to be extremely humble and extremely courageous in discovering his life story."

"What he has done is simply extraordinary. I never seen an individual in such despair facing the abyss and finality of his existence into transforming into a tour de force in serving the brain injury community. I have seen him save lives literally in front of my eyes ... which still astounds me ... yet I am not surprised by the outreach from elite sportspeople who seek his unique skills."

"Yet it is not the rich and famous that he has the greatest impact... it is the fallen human being who has left themselves for dead... he brings them back to life... and for that, we should have the utmost gratitude he has written this book.

This is his incredible work. His book is astonishingly useful & practical in the recovery of the human mind no matter what the circumstances.

Kudos"

- **Sir Marco Robinson,** #1 Bestselling Author, Top #2 Netflix Producer

"Dr. Brody Miller's *Brain Rescue* is a transformative guide for anyone seeking to reclaim their cognitive health and unlock the healing power of neuroplasticity. This book is an exceptional blend of science, personal triumph, and actionable tools that will leave readers inspired and empowered. With its clear, relatable narrative and practical advice, *Brain Rescue* deserves every one of its five stars."

"Dr. Miller's story is as gripping as it is inspiring. From his personal battles with brain injury, addiction, and devastating life choices, he emerges as a beacon of hope, proving that the brain can heal itself. He writes, "Recovering from a brain injury is truly like one big, scattered puzzle... you have to slowly put the pieces back together." This vulnerability invites readers to see their own struggles as surmountable challenges, not insurmountable obstacles."

"The heart of *Brain Rescue* lies in its exploration of neuroplasticity. Dr. Miller explains this complex concept in simple terms, describing it as "the ability of the brain and nervous system to change, heal, and adapt in response to our deepest beliefs, thoughts, emotions, actions, behaviors, and habits." This forms the foundation for the book's practical strategies, making it not just a compelling read but a manual for self-improvement."

"What truly sets *Brain Rescue* apart is its actionable content. From tools for enhancing memory and combating brain fog to strategies for managing emotional triggers, every chapter brims with advice readers can implement immediately. For example, in the chapter on memory recovery, Dr. Miller introduces exercises that simplify daily challenges, proving that "it isn't as difficult or complicated as you think, as long as you are willing to put in the time and effort."

"The book's emotional resonance is also a highlight. Dr. Miller's reflections on his darkest moments, such as his struggles with self-worth and his physical health, are balanced with stories of resilience and hope. He urges readers to embrace change, writing, "The ability to make different choices from yesterday is what separates us from the rest of the animal kingdom. Choose wisely. Change your choices, change your brain, change your energy, change your life!"

"*Brain Rescue* is not just a book; it's a call to action. Whether you're recovering from an injury, dealing with chronic stress, or simply striving for a sharper mind, this book provides the tools and inspiration needed to succeed. Its blend of personal anecdotes, scientific grounding, and practical advice ensures it will remain a go-to resource for readers long after they've turned the last page."

"If you're ready to take control of your brain health and transform your life, Dr. Miller's *Brain Rescue* is the perfect guide. This is more than a book—it's a lifeline, packed with hope and solutions for a brighter, healthier future."

- **Patrick K. Porter, Ph.D,** Author, Inventor of BrainTap
Dean of Brain-Based Medicine at Quantum University

"Dr. Brody pulls out all the tricks from under his sleeve to help brain injury survivors. He provides his readers with powerful strategies, techniques, and exercises backed by science to recover and overcome their struggles right now. The best part about the book is knowing Dr. Brody's brain injury story and realizing that he has led by example. You have so much to gain by reading his wisdom and applying the principles in this book. I highly recommend it to any TBI victim!"
-**Jorge Quintero,** NASM PT, Engineer, and Future Clinical Neuroscientist

"Dr. Brody Miller is a maverick when it comes to simplifying the complexities of the human brain and putting the neuro-puzzle pieces into fun and challenging strategies. A brilliant mind!"

- **Dr. Roman Velasquez,** CEO of Neuro Peak Performance

"Couldn't put it down!"

    -**Elizabeth Dimevska**, Entrepreneur, Courage Catalyst & Energy Activator Coach

"The information in this book can help set a solid foundation for those recovering from brain injury and concussion (mTBI)."

    - **Cavin Balaster** (Brain Injury Survivor & Thriver CEO of How to Feed-A-Brain)

© 2025 DR. BRODY MILLER

All rights reserved. No portion of this book or audiobook may be reproduced, stored in a retrieval system, or transmitted in any form or by any means—electronic, mechanical, photocopying, recording, scanning, or otherwise—without the prior written permission of the author or publisher, except for brief quotations used in critical reviews or scholarly articles.

The author, Dr. Brody Miller, asserts their moral right to be identified as the creator of this work in accordance with applicable intellectual property laws, including sections 77 and 78 of the Copyright, Designs, and Patents Act 1988.

All rights reserved. Unauthorized reproduction, distribution, or use of this material in any form is strictly prohibited and may result in legal action.

DISCLAIMER

The information provided in this book, on DrBrodymiller.com, or on affiliated websites is intended for informational and educational purposes only. It is not a substitute for professional medical advice, diagnosis, or treatment. Readers should not use the information contained in this book or on affiliated websites to diagnose or treat any medical condition or health concern.

Always seek the advice of a licensed healthcare professional regarding any medical condition or symptoms that require diagnosis or treatment. Never disregard professional medical advice or delay seeking it because of information presented in this book or on affiliated websites.

By using this book or associated websites, you acknowledge and agree that neither the author, Dr. Brody Miller, nor any affiliates, partners, or publishers are liable for any outcomes resulting from the application of the information provided. This includes, but is not limited to, direct, indirect, incidental, or consequential harm or damages.

No representations or warranties, express or implied, are made regarding the accuracy, completeness, or applicability of the information contained in this book or affiliated websites to your individual circumstances. Use of this material is at your own risk.

ISBN: 9798310707597

Cover esign by: Yasir Nadeem

*Dedicated to my amazing wife Rocio, mi pajarita más bonita del mundo.
Thank you deeply for believing in me when I didn't yet believe in myself.*

*To my loving parents, Lori and Thom Miller. Thank you for your
unwavering support, standing by me, and never giving up, through all of
the dark storms we have faced and overcome.*

To all my friends and family members, I love y'all.

*To the reader
Your recovery process is not always going to be an
easy process. There will be many highs and lows...
Like most people, you also have questions and doubts
I encourage you to give yourself lots of patience and compassion.
Trust in the process and the incredible ability of the brain to get better
over time*

CONTENTS

Who Is This Book For?	11
Introduction	13
Chapter One: Rewiring The Broken Circuit	23
Chapter Two: The Irony Of Head Injury	31
Chapter Three: Starting Your Recovery Journey	37
Chapter Four: The First Pillar: R Is For R.E.F.O.C.U.S	41
Chapter Five: The Second Pillar: E Is For E.N.G.A.G.E	77
Chapter Six: The Third Pillar: B Is For B.R.A.I.N	93
Chapter Seven: The Fourth Pillar: O Is For O.P.T.I.M.I.Z.E	111
Chapter Eight: The Fifth Pillar: U Is For U.N.L.E.A.S.H	145
Chapter Nine: The Sixth Pillar: N Is For N.E.X.U.S	167
Chapter Ten: The Seventh Pillar: D Is For D.E.D.I.C.A.T.E	179
Chapter Eleven: Brain Injury Warriors. "Stories Of Hope!"	199
Afterword	207
Bonus Chapter	213
Citations	223
About the Author	227

WHO IS THIS BOOK FOR?

I'll admit writing this is emotional for me. This book is for a version of myself I'll never forget. Speaking to the version that desperately needed love and didn't yet believe in his ability to heal. I was committed to getting better, but I didn't know how to build momentum. If you're reading this, you might feel that same sense of confusion, frustration, or fear right now. I've been there.

A QUICK HEADS-UP: Some parts of this book might be hard to hear or seem rather offensive. It is not my intention to make anyone feel bad about where they are in their recovery journey. I understand that brain injury comes in many forms, and there is no "one-size-fits-all solution. But if you're here, it's because you are ready for a change or a shift, and that's exactly what I'm going to help you achieve. This book is written for all the brave brain injury survivors dealing with the long-lasting effects of post-concussion syndrome or all the other many manifestations of brain injury. If you are navigating the challenges of life after an accident, you get how difficult it can be to reclaim your focus, your memory, your momentum, and your sense of normalcy. Even if you've experienced concussions before, the impact of this one may feel different, more severe, and more lasting.

If it's been months, and you're still battling with brain fog, memory lapses, and impulsiveness, while your relationships and professional goals seem to slip further out of your control, then you understand it can be hard to stay optimistic. You've probably tried many types of "self-improvement" before, but right now, you are at a crossroad. You want more clarity, more actionable steps, and real tools that can help you get back on track, not feeling isolated or abandoned by your friends and loved ones. You've tried lots of things, but nothing seems to work, or at least not for long. You're searching for a solution that goes beyond symptom management and dives deep into the root cause of your issues. This book will help you understand what's happening in your brain and how you can start recovering in a way that's practical, empowering, and specific to your unique needs. This isn't just theory. It's a proven approach grounded in both science and my own personal experience. The methods I share here helped me heal, and they've helped countless others do the same.

No need to feel lost anymore. The path to recovery starts with understanding, and this book will give you that clarity and the tools necessary to take control of your healing journey. As you read through the pages, you'll feel a renewed sense of empowerment. You'll learn actionable steps and hear real-life stories that show what's possible when you apply the right mindset and strategies.

Let's get started. This book will push you to face the deep part of you and take the necessary steps toward a successful recovery. I'll be with you every step of the way, because I know you can do this.

INTRODUCTION

"The Doctor with a Broken Brain"
How to Go from Foggy to Focused in 90 Days

> *"A Journey Of A Thousand Miles Begins With A Single Step"*
>
> — LAO TZU

Statistically speaking, I should be a dead man. But the universe had other plans for me.

Hi, I'm Dr. Brody, and I'm here to show you how to reclaim your memory, your focus, and your life, even if it feels like all hope is lost. My story isn't just about recovery, it's about resilience, rebirth, and the incredible power of the human brain to heal. I wasn't always known as "Dr. Brody." In the past, people labeled me as a drunk, punk, drug addict, and failure. However, today, I am a well-known brain rehabilitation specialist and an accredited Doctor with a PhD. I'm living proof that no matter how far you've fallen, it's possible to rebuild, and thrive. This is my wild story, from failures to freedom.

In 2013, I was a walking disaster. **One warm summer night outside of a dingy nightclub**, I found myself stumbling around, so drunk I could barely even stand. Liquid courage was pulsing through my veins, and I decided it was a good idea to pick a fight with a bouncer who was three times my size. The dude threw a vicious haymaker that knocked me out cold on the street. I was knocked completely unconscious for over 5 minutes, as everyone froze in shock as to what just happened. To add insult to injury, the whole incident was caught on camera and went viral on the internet. Seriously! A local news TV station broadcasted my lowest moment to the world, and eventually, **over 100,000 people had front-row tickets to me at my absolute worst.** I do not remember much from that time, but I do remember the shame and humiliation I felt as my parents watched the video. My dad took it especially hard as he responded in anger, saying, "I'm going to find this bastard and beat the sh*t out of him!" The months that followed were a blur of pain, regret, and suffocating darkness. I fell into a deep brain fog and stayed isolated in my house for months. The world was a blur as I felt completely numb to everyone and everything. My **memory** felt like a shattered mirror, pieces scattered so far that I could hardly remember who I was anymore. The depression was relentless and followed me everywhere like a black cloud. I vividly remember staring at myself in the mirror, hating my own reflection, and pulling out my hair, asking questions like, **"Why couldn't you have just died"**? Life was pain, and pain was life for me. This is when my reckless nature truly went into overdrive. My decision-making abilities became that of a 4-year-old child again. Deep down, I was crying out for help, but nothing was coming to save me. I wanted to feel something, really anything, to make me feel alive again.

So, I got into rock climbing and combined it with taking drugs, taunting death with every ascent, but at least I felt alive again. Eventually, I got a DUI, and my family sent me to a nine-month drug rehab program. I graduated the first stage and moved to a step-down program in Tucson, Arizona. I thought maybe, just maybe, that I was

Humpty Dumpty, and I could put all the pieces back together in my life again. **Recovering from a brain injury is like one big, scattered puzzle, with pieces thrown all over the place, that you have to slowly put back together.** However, I was doing relatively well until the day arrived which changed my life forever.

It was a hot sunny day, and I was speaking to my AA sponsor about the fourth step, to admit my deepest darkest secrets. And bam! Out of nowhere, I felt an immense burst of energy, like all my walls were closing in. My panicking body literally screamed out in sheer pain while my mind felt a deep sense of doom. **Was I dying?** I blacked out completely and awoke in a hospital bed. Doctors told me, "Mr. Miller, you just had three grand mal seizures." **Oh great.** Doctors ordered a brain scan and discovered a 2.5 cm cavernous malformation (essentially a benign brain tumor) in my left frontal lobe that was leaking blood into my brain. That was the culprit that was causing the seizures. A few months later, neurosurgeons cut open my brain and removed the malformation. Was I on the right path, finally? Sadly, no.

Just three days after the surgery, I suffered another horrific series of seizures and was rushed back to the hospital. The ordeal escalated as I was airlifted by helicopter to a hospital in Phoenix. Thankfully, it turned out to not be life-threatening, but it was an incredibly frightening time for all of us. Adding to the stress, I realized how broken the medical system was when my family was hit with a **staggering bill of over $80,000** for the helicopter ride and treatment.

The next few years, things did not improve; in fact, they worsened. I continued to have 3 grand mal seizures a month, hitting my head, bloodying my nose, and experiencing more concussions. Not exactly the best thing for brain health. They filled me up with all kinds of meds. Anti-depressants, anti-psychotics, anti-seizure meds etc.... I ended having such a violent reaction to Keppra, an anti-seizure medication, that I started feeling homicidal. Have you ever felt that eerie feeling? Being suicidal is one thing, but to have the urge and drive to kill another person is equally as scary. I was acting insane, well I was insane, and so I was taken to a mental institution for a night. The AA wisdom "Hospitals, Jails, and Mental Institutions" really rang true to me. There was only one ugly horseman left, and that was death.

I ended up developing horrific chronic nerve pain in both of my forearms that was **so bad that I couldn't even do a single pushup** without excruciating pain. My loving family and I constantly went from one medical professional to the next, test after test, desperately searching for answers, but we only received confused looks, and blank stares back from the doctors.

Maybe you've been there, or somewhere like it. Perhaps you're struggling with brain fog, memory lapses, or a sense that life as you knew it is slipping through your fingers. I see you. I know the questions that keep you up at night. Will I ever feel normal again? Can I get my life back. The answer is a resounding YES. This book is proof.

The truth is, **your brain is not broken,** as a matter of fact, **it's capable of incredible healing. Neuroplasticity, the science of change, is the key to rewriting your brain's story.** It's not just theory; it's the very thing that saved my life. For those of you, who may not know, neuroplasticity is the ability of the brain and nervous system to change, heal, and adapt in response to our deepest beliefs, thoughts, emotions, actions, behaviors, and habits.

The healthcare system doesn't want you to believe this. They want you to be reliant on their opinions and authority. But they are dead wrong! Neuroplasticity gave me hope in my darkest hours. I'm not the only one who has witnessed the power of neuroplasticity. Friends of mine have defied the odds, recovering from injuries like diffuse axonal injury, one of the most severe forms of brain trauma. 90% of people diagnosed with this from injury never emerge from a minimally conscious state. They, too, were told their futures were bleak. And they, too, proved the experts wrong. What I spoke of above is why I call myself the **Doctor who used to have a "Broken Brain."** Because at the time of my injury, doctors told me I had a broken brain, and now, ironically, I am a Doctor with his PhD! **How ironic!** I am living proof that you can make a comeback with your brain health, regardless of how bad it seems. Regardless of what a whitey, tidy, underwear-wearing doctor tells you.

Listen, life is not easy for anyone. I've hit rock bottom in life several times now. The first was having seizures in hospitals, and the second time when I had to serve a 60-day jail sentence for my several DUIs. Mental health issues are very real and something we all need to seriously focus on taking more care of. But no matter how far you fall, I promise you can always make the **CHOICE** to change your life for the better. The ability to make different choices from yesterday is what separates us from the rest of the animal kingdom. **Choose wisely.**

And best of all, that's **just the tip of the iceberg!** Because it is just a sneak preview of the amazing wisdom of what is to come in this book.

Why does this book focus on memory? And what will you accomplish from reading the book?

Memory is the foundation of who we are. I didn't fully grasp it's importance until I lost mine after the bouncer incident. My short-term memory was so poor that I was forgetting virtually everything, like where my wallet was or what was spoken of in recent conversations. **This book is called "Brain Rescue" because that is exactly what it is designed to do: Rescue Your Brain!** My mission is to share the tools I wish I had after my injuries. Memory is also one of the most complex and misunderstood phenomena in the ENTIRE UNIVERSE. But it is one of the most essential aspects of living a healthy and happy life. It is my goal to demystify memory, break it down into actionable steps and prove to you that you can get your memory back and sharper than ever before, even after a brain injury or multiple concussions. This can be accomplished without having to go to countless doctor's visits, take medications with horrific side effects, undergo risky surgeries, and spend hundreds of thousands of dollars! I am here to show you that it isn't as difficult or complicated as you think as long as you are willing to put in the time and effort.

If you're skeptical, good! You should be! The traditional medical system is broken, and sadly, there are more scams than ever before in these modern times of AI, where it is difficult to decipher real from fake.

The Hard Questions

If you've picked up this book, whether it's for a loved one or yourself, you're likely grappling with painful questions like:

- Why do I still have brain fog months after my injury? Shouldn't I be feeling better by now?
- Will my memory ever come back, or is this something I'll have to live with forever?
- How do I know if my brain is healing or just getting worse over time?
- Could the memory loss and damage from my injury be irreversible?
- Am I at a higher risk for developing Parkinson's, Alzheimer's or other awful brain diseases?

Or you may be feeling....

- A sense of guilt and shame for using your family's money and time for your recovery.
- Sick and tired of others feeling pity for you and your situation.
- Exhausted. It's difficult to find the motivation to just get out of bed on some days.
- Overwhelmed and distracted, because it's difficult to control your focus at all!

- Or you are just sick and tired of being clucking sick and tired!

If you identify with one or more of the above, then this book is **DEFINITELY** for you. As you probably know, recovering from a brain injury is HARD! It's a lot of work! But do you know what's even more difficult? Hoping and praying for a different result without taking the steps needed to create change.

Your brain is an incredible organ, designed for survival and energy conservation. But make no mistake about it. **We will always do more to avoid pain than to create pleasure.**

Brain injuries catapult us into a chronic state of survival. To move away from pain and discomfort, we tend to think about pain and discomfort!

This is a huge trap! In recovery, it is so important that we focus our attention and energy on what we **DO WANT** vs What We Don't Want! Think of recovery like climbing up a slow, icy, dangerous mountain. There will be obstacles and setbacks, no doubt. But it will do you absolutely o good to focus on the obstacles. It's all about refocusing on where you do want to go vs where you don't want to go on the mountain. Think of me like a Sherpa, helping guide you up the mountain and giving you tips. But ultimately, it is up to you to climb the mountain.

So, as you read every word of this page, I will address those questions in my highest understanding of the truth. But not just from studying textbooks (cough, like most doctors) but from a place of experience.

Now, pay close attention!

Throughout This Guide You Will Discover:

- **Scientific Ideas Simplified**: Easy-to-understand explanations of brain health, neuroplasticity, and how to rewire your brain for a better memory.

- **A Clear, Easy to Follow 90-Day Blueprint**: Proven guidance on how to reclaim your memory, focus, and cognitive abilities after a concussion or brain injury, by using the **R.E.B.O.U.N.D. Method.**

- **Real Stories of Hope (Third Party Hero's Journey)**: Inspirational stories from friends, clients, and colleagues who have made remarkable comebacks from severe brain injuries. This is to expand your mind to what is truly possible when you put in the work.

In **Brain Rescue**, I am going to cover the most relevant and up-to-date neuro-scientific information about **memory** after a head injury, but I will also cover it from an energetic standpoint. Because, at the end of the day, as Nickola Tesla said, everything in the universe is made up of "energy, frequency, and vibration." But do not worry; this book is made for both advanced and beginners alike. If you begin to understand the **five principles of neuroplasticity** and, most importantly, apply them to your daily life, you will be well on your way to a successful recovery.

Thank you for your attention, Warriors. Ultimately, this book is written to give you all the tools I wish I had at the time of my injury so that you don't have to go through all of the unnecessary pain and hard lessons. **This is your moment.** No more sitting back, waiting, or wondering when you'll get better. Right here, right now, you need to understand that your brain is begging for you to step up. You've been knocked down by this concussion, but here's the thing. Doctors, old friends, and family are probably underestimating you. Your brain has the power to rebuild, to get stronger, and to come back with an entirely new perspective on life. But you've got to own that process. If you struggle with focus and concentration and are overwhelmed, I highly recommend that you take it easy and digest this book at your own pace, whatever that may look like for you. Bit by bit it will add up to a lot!

Change your thoughts, change your choices, change your energy, change your life!

~Dr. Brody

CHAPTER ONE: REWIRING THE BROKEN CIRCUIT

The Beginners Guide to Memory Recovery

Imagine waking up one morning, and the world around you feels strangely unfamiliar. You know the faces and voices of your loved ones, but every detail, their laughs, the memories you've shared, feels blurred and almost unreachable. Now imagine each day slipping further from your grasp as if your life is written in sand, constantly swept away by the tide.

For millions who've suffered head injuries, this isn't a nightmare.... It's their reality.

It doesn't take a **neuroscience degree** from Stanford to realize that the brain is very important. If you get shot in the head, you're dead! Even though most people know that intuitively, why, after a concussion or brain injury, are they told to just "wait" or shake it off?"

Sadly, we can reminisce on the negative impact repetitive head trauma had upon athletes like Muhammad Ali, Junior Seau, Antonio Brown, Aaron Hernandez, the list goes on. May their downfalls not go in vain. **There is absolutely nothing in this world is more important than your brain health! Not even 100's of millions of dollars!** Have you noticed the trend of more and more combat sports fighters looking to retire from their professions at a very young age. Star athletes like Paul Rosas Jr. and Gervonta Davis have come to realize **undeniable truth! Bad brain health equals bad memory and poor quality of life.**

Memory isn't just a nice ability; it's our life, it's our very essence. As humans, we tend to overlook the importance of the things we cannot see. Brain injury is called the "Invisible Epidemic" for this very reason. Connections suffer, families are impacted financially, and relationships are devastated mentally and emotionally. The average concussion takes an impact of 95 g's (gravity) force to create, **but regardless of the level of severity, head injuries** should **ALWAYS** be taken very **seriously**. They happen repetitively in sports like soccer and rugby, where blows may not be as severe but add up due to their consistent nature. Like anything else in life, both how intense an event is and how many times it happens really matters.

Look at it this way…When you experience a head injury, your brain **violently jolts** back and forth rapidly. The rapid **acceleration** and **deceleration** causes **stretching**, **shearing**, and **tearing** to the connecting tissues of the brain called axons. Axons connect one neuron (brain cell) to another. When they get stretched out, the brain cannot communicate the way it needs to from one area to the next. Most concussions impact the front, bottom, and side areas of the brain.

The result? A whole host of potential symptoms and issues.

SHOCKING MISCONCEPTIONS ABOUT BRAIN INJURIES

A common **misconception** is brain injuries only happen from hitting your head. That's not true. There are many types of brain injuries. For example, chemical brain injuries can happen from drug use or certain medications, and viral brain injuries can come from infections like COVID-19 or bacteria. There are also **brain injuries** that happen when the brain doesn't get enough oxygen, like after a stroke or a near-drowning event, and toxic brain injuries from harmful **chemicals** in the body.

And that's not all. Other forms of brain injuries include degenerative diseases such as Alzheimer's that slowly damage the brain; tumor-related injuries that put pressure on brain tissue; and vascular injuries, like strokes, which happen when blood flow to the brain is blocked.

Isn't it fair then to say that every single brain injury is truly unique?

For the sake of this book, we are going to focus on head injuries and concussions that occur from an external force and impact. However, just know that the science-backed tools provided in the book will be helpful for a wide variety of brain injuries.

Head injuries are **devastating**, especially to **memory**. Sometimes, they wipe out the ability to remember what happened yesterday; other times, they steal pieces of who we once were. In most cases, both short-term and long-term memories are negatively affected, leaving people feeling fragmented, as if pieces of their own lives are just out of reach.

The numbers are startling: over 65% of concussions strike the front of the skull. That's where the **"frontal lobe"—the commander of our minds**—lives. The **frontal lobe** isn't just another part of the brain; it's the general, the leader, the president, shaping our identity, personality, focus, decision-making, and willpower. It's where we imagine our future and draw from our past. When damaged, the effects can unravel the very core of who we are.

I know this firsthand. When I was hit by that bouncer, it was as if any filter my young brain had was ripped away. I became impulsive, **reckless**, and driven by **urges I could barely control.** Rock climbing while intoxicated, venturing into dangerous areas in Central America to buy drugs, and even getting arrested in the Dominican Republic—these weren't just moments of poor judgment. They were signs of a much deeper problem. My mood swings became **violent** and unpredictable, and each day was a fresh hell of anxiety and sleepless nights. I was living in a nightmare, and the worst part was I couldn't wake myself up!

Let me be a bit more specific. When the frontal lobe is damaged, it causes **memory issues**, especially with short-term memory. That explains why many people who have suffered from a brain injury can vividly remember significant events in their life story but struggle to recall where they put their keys or what they spoke about in a recent conversation. Think about it: if memory shapes every single choice we make, how can we understand it—and reclaim it—when it starts to slip away?

Before we get into the how-to, let's explore what memory truly is. **Memory is everything!** It's not just a tool; it's the foundation of our entire quality of life! It sets the context for everything we know, everything we feel, and everything we hope for. Meaning that only by understanding **who we are**, where we have come from, and where we are currently, can we frame what we want to do in the next moments, the next days, the next years, and the rest of our lives. Memory is the brain's way of **acquiring, storing, organizing, and retrieving** information. Imagine it like a computer: encoding is like typing in the information, consolidation is saving it, storage is keeping it safe in the brain, and retrieval is pulling it up when you need it. Scientifically, memory is a puzzle we still haven't completely solved! Yet, understanding these basic **mechanics** has been essential in my own journey of recovery. As you go through this chapter, you'll see that memory isn't just a process; it's deeply personal, connected to everything we value and strive for.

So, to break it down scientifically, there are **3 main forms of memory**. Short term memory, working memory and long-term memory.

1. **Short-Term Memory (Passive)**

- **Timing:** Typically lasts for about 15-30 seconds.
- **Capacity:** Most humans can remember, on average, 5-9 bits of information at a time.
- **Example:** Remembering someone's phone number for a few seconds without writing it down. If you don't repeat it quickly, you'll forget it in about 15-30 seconds.

2. **Working (Active) Memory:**

- **Timing:** Temporary storage, used at the moment.
- **Capacity:** Like short-term memory, it can hold about 5-9 items. However, it works as long as you are ACTIVELY using it.
- **Example:** Doing math in your head or remembering directions while walking.

3. **Long-Term Memory.**

- **Timing:** Days, Months, Years, Decades.
- **Capacity:** Practically Limitless.
- **Example:** Remembering exactly where you were and what you were doing on 9/11 after the Twin Towers fell.

The Bottom Line

- **Short-term memory** holds memories briefly.
- **Working memory** keeps information in play as long as you're actively using it.
- **Long-term memory** stores what your brain believes is the most important information, for better or for worse.

Remember... Learning is memory in action! As you read each word of this page, you are forming new neural connections, new associations and memories! How remarkable is that?

I could go on about the different types of **memory**—like declarative memories, which include episodic and semantic memory, and non-declarative memories, such as procedural, innate, and emotional memory—but I'll save that for another part of this book. At the end, there will be a bonus chapter just for all you seekers who want to dive deeper into the mechanics of memory.

But for now, let's keep it practical. After all, this book is written for all you **Badass Brain Recovery Warriors!** So now that we've covered **what memory** is, let's move into the "**why.**"

REBUILDING YOUR MEMORY IS IMPORTANT

Once again **memory** *is* everything! Without memory, life would be completely without meaning. You wouldn't remember your favorite moments, your friends, or even your own story. Memories become super meaningful **ONLY** because of the emotions we attach to them.

Think about this: AI can remember facts, and even learn to some extent, but without emotions, that memory has no weight, no significance. Human memory is different, it's deeply **meaningful** and **interconnected.** Therefore, improving one form of memory strengthens others.

For example, when you work on strengthening your episodic memory (memory for events), you also boost your semantic memory (memory for facts). It's all interconnected!

Bear with me because I'm going to briefly teach how the brain stores memories holistically. Sounds are stored in the temporal lobe, located near the ears, while visual memories are stored in the occipital lobe at the back of the brain. Short-term and working memories rely on the prefrontal cortex. Sensory memories, like touch are processed in the somatosensory cortex, and the limbic system stores memories of smells, closely linked to our emotional experiences. Each of these regions plays a vital role in maintaining the complex web of connec-tions that shape our memories and our ability to recall them. You may be asking, ughh, whatsup DOC?

Why does this matter? Because it proves that memory is holistic and that memories are not only stored in one part of the brain.

We know this because damage to these different areas of the brain directly affect how well certain memories and specific brain regions function. But here's something important to remember. Memory doesn't just reside in the brain, it's stored in the entire nervous system, connecting every part of who we are. I believe deep down that every single cell of human body has it's own intelligence and ability to learn and store memories.

The big takeaway? Improving your memory is like sharpening a tool. The more you practice, the stronger and more effective your memory becomes. Every small improvement you make strengthens your foundation, so keep learning, keep pushing forward, and remember: each step you take is a victory on your journey toward a sharper mind and a fuller life. I can't stress this enough! **Practice does not make perfection like you have been told. Practice makes progress!** And eventually they become permanent or automatic networks in the brain.

Now that you have a better understanding of memory, there's just one more vital chapter to set the stage before we dive into the actionable strategies of the **7-Step R.E.B.O.U.N.D. Method.**

I urge you not to skip ahead, yet. This next short chapter will provide the essential insights and tools you'll need to fully harness the power of this transformative recovery framework.

Ready to start working on your memory? Get your free 15 Mind Gym Exercises. By visiting www.dr-bro.com/vipbrainrescue or scan the QR code below.

CHAPTER TWO: THE IRONY OF HEAD INJURY

How Your Heart Holds the Key to Brain Health

It's almost absurd to claim that the key to **memory recovery starts in the heart?** Memory is stored in the brain, right? After a head injury, it's only natural to think that all the healing should be aimed at the brain. And yet, there's a surprising twist here. By focusing on the heart, you'll not only enhance your brain's function, but also create a **foundation** for holistic recovery. And that's not all. **Did you know that it is a scientific fact that the heart sends more information to the brain than the brain does to the heart?** Astonishing, isn't it? The heart produces more energy than any other organ by far! Beyond just pumping blood, the heart is constantly in communication with the brain through electrical, hormonal, and biochemical signals. In fact, research shows that when the heart maintains the special frequency of 0.1 Hz when it creates waves that harmonize it with the brain. This beautiful connection is called 'heart-brain coherence', helping the mind and body work together in harmony.[1]

And that's not all!

Science shows that the heart sends signals to the brain not only through nerve pathways but also through its powerful electromagnetic field, which can shift mental states and affect healing. This heart-brain communication speeds up and helps repair neural pathways damaged by head trauma. The heart's magnetic field is the strongest field within the human body.

And YES! There is neuroplasticity in the heart as well. Most people have a huge misunderstanding that neuroplasticity is only in the brain. That's simply not true!

Neuroplasticity, once again, is the ability of the brain, heart, and nervous system to change, heal and adapt over time in response to everything we do. Your heart, like your brain has an incredible ability to adapt and change.

What if I told you, by tapping into this 'heart neuroplasticity' you will supercharge your recovery? What if by improving the connection between your brain and your heart, you would improve memory, resilience, and your health more than you could ever imagine? I'm here to inform you that this is not only possible, but probable, if you learn and embody what I am about to teach you.

The heart is our emotional center, meaning it is the core of all our emotions. And what are emotions? They are just simply energy in motion! When we feel elevated emotions like **appreciation, love, gratitude care, and inspiration**, our heart shows measurable changes in heart rate, heart rate variability and coherence. By nature, these are healing energies to our psychology (mind), neurology (brain), biology (body) and spirit (soul).

But when we are feeling negative emotions like **frustration, anxiety, guilt, shame, agitation or fear**, there are noticeable negative changes in our health, biology, and wellbeing. The heart truly is the key to our health and overall performance.

Check out this amazing research image, credit of the **Heart Math Institute,** to get a better understanding of what I am referring of.

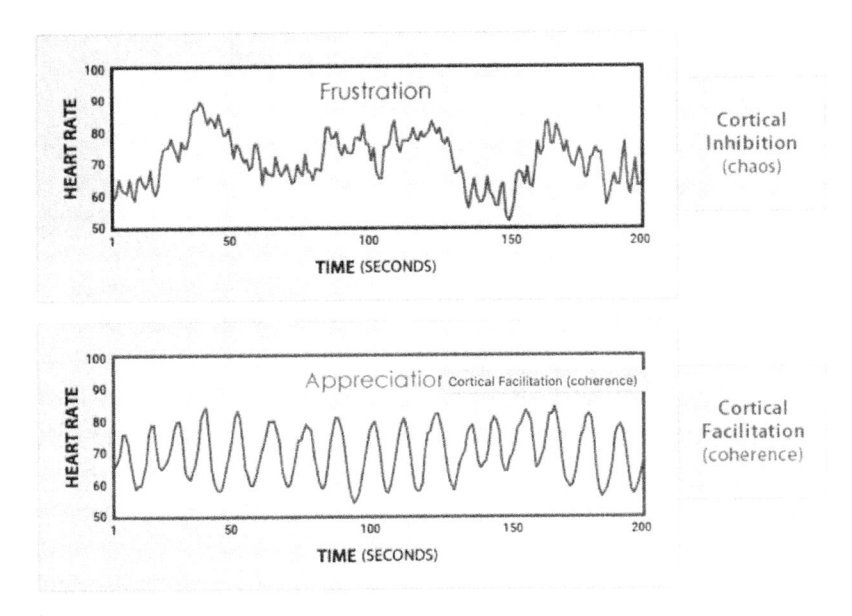

[Frustration heart rate graph — Cortical Inhibition (chaos)]

[Appreciation heart rate graph — Cortical Facilitation (coherence)]

Patterns of the HRV waveforms are clearly different.

Now, let's look at three extremely important health metrics I pay the most attention to in the work I do with my patients. Better yet, we will break them down as simply as we can.

Know that there are three very important health statistics (metrics) for the heart. Heart rate, heart rate variability (HRV), and coherence. While they may sound similar, each plays a unique and important role.

1. **Heart Rate:** This is the number of times your heart beats per minute. A lower resting heart rate generally means a healthier heart.

2. **Heart Rate Variability (HRV):** HRV shows the difference (variation) in time between heartbeats. A higher HRV means your body handles stress better, is more resilient and recovers well. A lower HRV means it's harder for your body to manage the effects of stress.

3. **Coherence:** Coherence occurs when the heart, mind, and emotions are in sync. Positive emotions like gratitude and love create a smooth, orderly heart rhythm, enhancing both heart and brain function. Incoherent emotions like frustration or fear do the opposite.

These three health markers are very important to improve after a head injury because they directly affect influence with how well you deal with stress and how resilient you are. When you experience a head injury it is a HUGE stressor to the brain and nervous system. So, a head injury is essentially a disruption in the brain's safety and understanding of the world. You are put into a long-lasting survival mode. You get knocked out of a state of balance and put into a state of DIS-EASE. Nothing is EASY and even the basics become more difficult. The third metric, coherence is honestly the most underrated health statistic I have ever encountered! I believe if people knew how to create more coherence, then there would be a significant decrease in chronic illness.

But don't take my word for it. Practice this exercise at the bottom of the chapter every day for the next few weeks, and you will know exactly what I am talking about!

Healing the old wounds of our heart is a must. **Recovery starts with courage and forgiveness.** We must shed our old wounds, accept our past and what happened, and begin to take baby steps in the direction that we want to each and every day!

This is a daily practice and just like anything in life, the more you practice something the better you get. Let's say you wanted to become a master breadmaker. Do you think the very first time you ever cooked bread it would come out perfectly crisp, tasting good?

NOPE.

That's why I want you to practice talking to your heart just like a good friend.

Heal your heart, heal your life.

Action Step! Brain and Heart Coherence in Three Steps

1. Close your eyes and gently place your hand over your heart.
2. Start to breathe a little slower and deeper than usual, with slightly longer exhales than inhales. Perhaps for the count of 4 seconds in and 6 seconds out. (Do not force your breathing pattern. Go at a pace of a natural rhythm that works for you)
3. Focus on a regenerative emotion, like love, peace or gratitude. If you find your mind wandering, that's ok, just refocus on a restorative feeling.

Step Into the VIP Circle! Get access to discounts, early offers, and free tools to sharpen your mind. **Scan the QR code or visit www.dr-bro.com/vipbrainrescue**

CHAPTER THREE: STARTING YOUR RECOVERY JOURNEY

The **R.E.B.O.U.N.D. Method** is a handy acronym and compilation of the most effective practices I've discovered through the thousands of hours I have dedicated to researching the brain. It's what I've seen work best with my patients, but equally important, it was developed through my trials and tribulations in my recovery journey. Unlike most healthcare practitioners out there, my methods are truly based upon my experiences instead of something that was simply read in a book.

This **90-day blueprint** was created with the scientific knowledge that it takes, on average, **60 to 254 days** to create an automatic habit, with somewhere around the 66-day mark being the sweet spot for most people.[2] As you read each word of this page, ask yourself this very important question. **What is the true value of a memory recovery blueprint?** A blueprint that eliminates the guesswork and leads to predictable results? That's the opportunity I am giving you with the R.E.B.O.U.N.D. method. Here are 7 Steps of this proven process.

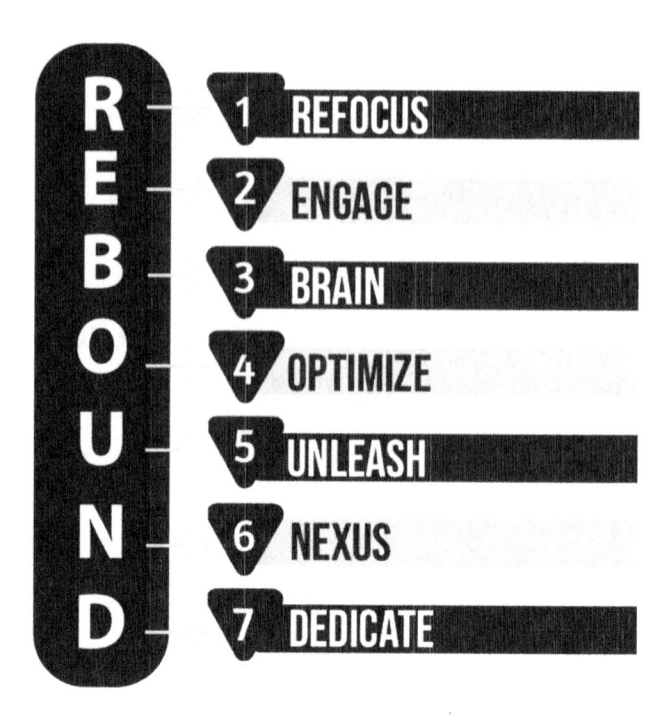

```
R ──┐  1 REFOCUS
E ──┤  2 ENGAGE
B ──┤  3 BRAIN
O ──┤  4 OPTIMIZE
U ──┤  5 UNLEASH
N ──┤  6 NEXUS
D ──┘  7 DEDICATE
```

R – R.E.F.O.C.U.S: *Refocus your energy. Ground your recovery with a rock-solid foundation through rest, nutrition, movement, and supplementation. This section builds a baseline for strength and resilience in the critical early stages.*

E- E.N.G.A.G.E: *Engage powerful pathways to long-term brain change, harnessing gratitude, energy, exercise and nitric oxide breathing to fuel both immediate progress and long term neuroplastic potential.*

B- B.R.A.I.N: *Master the 5 core principles of neuroplasticity—breath, repetition association, intensity, and novelty—to create transformative and lasting brain changes you can rely on.*

O- O.P.T.I.M.I.Z.E: *Optimize your recovery to the next level with a cutting-edge brain optimization system that sharpens focus, processing, and timing to exceed your own cognitive goals.*

U- U.N.L.E.A.S.H: *Unleash your true power. Break through mental limits* *by tapping into the subconscious, activating the vagus nerve, and integrating super learning techniques to unleash unprecedented potential.*

N- N.E.X.U.S: Unlock the mysteries of reality using principles of quantum physics, where entanglement, energy fields, and superposition empower you to shape your world.

D- D.E.D.I.C.A.T.E: Commit fiercely to lifelong growth: strengthen your identity, align your conscious and subconscious, and develop cognitive flexibility to maintain an empowered recovery journey.

The **R.E.B.O.U.N.D. Method** is a step-up process. Meaning that depending on where you are in your recovery journey, we will either speed up or slow down because every brain is different.

Ready to start your recovery journey today? Scan now to join the VIP priority list and receive your free memory-boosting exercises.

CHAPTER FOUR: THE FIRST PILLAR: R IS FOR R.E.F.O.C.U.S

The first stage **R.E.F.O.C.U.S.** is all about setting a solid foundation for an empowered recovery. Within each pillar are also mini pillars to make this a step-by-step guide.

THE FIRST STEP IS R FOR REST:

> *"Sleep Is The Single Most Effective Thing We Can Do To Reset Our Brain Health Each Day"*
>
> — DR. MATTHEW WALKER

Think of a **head injury** the same way you would view a sprained ankle or a broken arm. How do you typically handle those kinds of injuries? By giving them **REST.** The challenge with a brain injury is understanding what "resting" the brain actually means. Jumping straight back into work, school, or any demanding mental or physical activities is like trying to run on a sprained ankle. It can hinder the healing process. Keep in mind that your brain requires **TONS of energy** to fully recover.

Let's be real. **Rest isn't a luxury. Every dog, cat, lion, lizard, shark, mammal, and bear are dependent on it at a deep biological level.** Even a Warrior recovering from battle needs it. And you are a true Warrior because brain injury is a real son of a bi*ch that very few people really understand! That's because they have never had to deal with it.

If you're struggling to sleep, I've been there myself. After my injury, I battled severe sleep deprivation that left me feeling broken. I didn't just lose sleep; I lost my sense of peace and clarity. **Navy SEALs** I have interviewed have told me that sleep deprivation is a torture tool commonly used in the military, and I can understand why.

Referring back to the main point, we all can agree that rest is an essential part of living a healthy life and restoring health. Many people are burning themselves out thinking they can hustle their way through recovery. It doesn't work like that. **Prioritizing rest is non-negotiable.** And it provides you a foundation of your health. Without it, your brain doesn't stand a chance at healing. Your neurons? They need time to repair, rebuild, and recharge. In fact, sleep is bar-none the most important part of memory consolidation (the ability to form new memories).

We all know that after you experience a concussion, you need more rest than normal. Most people are still told to sleep it off. I see it differently. Do you need lots of rest? Yes. But you also need activity to get blood flow going. Rest alone will not give you the results.

Concussions interrupt sleep patterns for many reasons: the headaches, the mood swings, the restlessness. It's like trying to sleep on a shaky, broken foundation. Let me explain...

When we go to sleep, **our brain's glymphatic system** (the "G" standing for glial cells) is hard at work cleaning out toxins that accumulate during the day. Imagine your brain as a bustling city. Throughout the day, trash piles up from all the activities, decisions, and learning you do. The glymphatic system is like the city's waste management crew, clearing out the debris while you sleep. It's not glamorous, but it's essential for keeping the city running smoothly.

But here's the catch... Imagine if that city's plumbing and waste systems were clogged or broken. The trash would pile up, causing chaos and impacting every part of the city's functioning. That's what happens in your brain after a head injury. The glymphatic system can't do its job the way it needs to.[3]

Toxins build up, creating a ripple effect that can impair memory, mood, focus, and overall healing. This is why sleep is so critical—not just any sleep, but high-quality, restorative sleep. Without it, your brain can't clean, repair, or recharge. And that's where my desire comes in. My goal is to help you establish a consistent sleeping routine and practice good sleep hygiene.

These two sleep strategies work together to rebuild your brain's 'waste system' and restore the natural rhythms essential for healing and thriving. The tips in the following section aim to help you establish a consistent sleep routine and practice good sleep hygiene, both of which are critical foundations for supporting sleep during early recovery.

Sleep Hygiene: The Foundation of Recovery

Good sleep is the cornerstone of brain health and recovery. Let's break it down into two crucial aspects: **routine** and **hygiene**.

1. Establish a Consistent Sleep Routine

Life thrives on patterns. The sun rises and sets, seasons shift predictably, and the human body functions best with consistent rhythms. Sleep is no exception. A regular sleep schedule trains your brain and body to anticipate rest, making it a habit that feels natural and automatic over time.

Here's my approach: I adhere to the "9-to-5" rule—not for work, but for sleep. I prioritize 8–9 hours nightly to give my brain the time it needs to repair, consolidate memories, and recharge.

Morning sunlight is another game-changer. Dr. Andrew Huberman's research highlights how exposure to morning light resets your **circadian rhythm** (your body's internal clock) that regulates sleep and wake cycles. For example, when traveling across time zones, like from New York to Bangkok, your circadian rhythm might take a week to adjust. Morning sunlight can speed up this process, aligning your internal clock with local time.

2. Optimize Sleep Hygiene

Sleep hygiene is about crafting the perfect environment and habits for restful sleep. Here are my top tips:

- **Power Down Early:** Stop working and scrolling social media at least an hour before bed. Blue light disrupts melatonin production, the hormone essential for sleep.
- **Create Complete Darkness:** Use blackout curtains to make your room pitch black. Darkness signals the pineal gland to release melatonin.
- **Eliminate Noise Pollution:** Invest in a white noise machine or earplugs to block disruptive sounds.
- **Keep It Cool:** The ideal sleep temperature is 65–70°F (18–21°C). Can't cool your room? Try a cold shower or an ice bath before bed—it's worth the effort.

Sleep deprivation can wreak havoc on your brain. Studies show that sleep-deprived individuals perform cognitively like someone legally drunk. Severe deprivation can even cause hallucinations. Simply put, **recovery without rest is impossible.**

If air conditioning isn't available, there are still effective ways to cool down for better sleep. Take a cold shower before bed or fill your bathtub with ice bags from the store to create an ice bath. While this may sound intense, the investment is well worth it, especially when you understand the critical role sleep plays in recovery.

Sleep deprivation is devastating for brain health. Research shows that even moderate sleep loss can impair your cognitive abilities to the level of being legally drunk. [4] Go without sleep for several days, and you may begin to hallucinate. That's why prioritizing sleep is *non-negotiable*, especially in early recovery. By consistently applying these strategies, you'll give your brain the rest it needs to heal, improve memory, and reduce brain fog. Recovery without rest is simply impossible. For extra insight, consider investing in a wearable like the Oura Ring. It can help you track your sleep quality, identify helpful habits, and eliminate disruptions, empowering you to fine-tune your routine and optimize your recovery.

7 Tips for Sleeping Like A Baby Again Even After A Head Injury

1. **Create Your Sacred Cave.** Make the room chilly, dark, and soundproof as possible, 64-68 degrees. Wear an eye mask and earplugs if necessary. Make your bedroom Sacred. For Sex and Sleeping ONLY.
2. **Get Morning and Evening Sunlight.** Get some sunlight early in the morning and in the evening. Natural light helps reset your internal clock (circadian rhythm), making it easier to fall asleep and wake up at the right time!
3. **Be Consistent.** Make sure to go to bed and wake up around the same time every day! Be strict at first to establish the pattern, but afterwards it will get easier.
4. **Cut the C.R.A.P.** – Carbonated drinks, refined sugars, added colors, and processed sugars.
5. **Add Background Sounds!** Adding background noises like white noise, nature sounds, hypnosis tapes or calming instrumentals can really help you sleep better.

6. **Try Meditation or Prayer.** Meditating before bed can seriously improve your sleep quality and reduce anxiety. Even just 5 minutes of meditation visualization or mindful prayer can help calm your brain, ease your mind, switch on your parasympathetic nervous system (rest and digest) and get you ready for a deep sleep.
7. **Take GABA, Theanine, and Ashwagandha for Extra Support.** These natural supplements can really help calm your nervous system. The best part is they are all non-addictive! If you need a little help, they can help you relax, reduce anxiety, and make it easier to fall into a restful sleep.

THE SECOND STEP IS E FOR EXERCISE:

> *"Nothing Speeds Brain Atrophy More Than Being Immobilized In The Same Environment"*
>
> — NORMAN DOIDGE

Mr. Doidge, one of the grandfathers of modern-day neuroplasticity, is trying to tell you something. He is saying that there is **NOTHING** more **DESTRUCTIVE** to **brain health** than the **LACK of movement** and **staying in the SAME environment.** In other words, nothing is more **toxic** to brain health than **stagnation.**

Damn! I wish someone had told me that! Because after my brain injury, I did the opposite—I sat in darkness, isolated, while my brain practically cried out for stimulation, for oxygen, and for life. Yes, rest has its place, but if you're not willing to move, you're really holding yourself back. **We need to GET YOU MOVING!** Movement is medicine, movement is life! If you desire an empowered recovery, but you're not willing to move your body, you are really screwing up! Your brain needs **oxygen,** it needs **blood flow,** and that's only going to happen if you consistently move! There are many myths about how to care for your brain after you experience a brain injury. I will address three common ones now.

3 Harmful Myths About Exercise And Head Injuries

Myth #1: "Just Rest It Off...."

The common recommendation after a concussion is to just wait it off and rest. **It is important to rest, I'm not denying that!** But, I would say that it is equally important to get moving in your recovery. We want to get you moving in a way that is truly empowering and fun.

More rest is necessary in the early stages, but too much rest without any movement can actually slow your recovery. Movement stimulates the brain and accelerates the healing process. Movement is medicine, and without it, we're allowing stagnation to take over—robbing our brains of the life, oxygen, and stimulation they need to rebuild and thrive.

BDNF and GDNF

Exercise is like **magic** for your brain. The science is extremely compelling. It helps your body make a special protein called **BDNF (Brain-Derived Neurotrophic Factor)**. Think of BDNF as "**brain fertilizer**" that helps your brain stay healthy and grow stronger by building better connections between brain cells. But that's not all! Exercise also boosts something called **GDNF (Glial Cell-Derived Neurotrophic Factor)**. **GDNF** comes from **glial cells**, which are like your brain's support team. While brain cells are the messengers that send signals in your brain, glial cells make sure those messengers have everything they need to do their job, like keeping them protected and energized. GDNF helps these neurons heal and stay strong, which is super important for mood and **memory**.[5] Did you know there are twice as many glial cells as there are brain cells? However, both cell forms are important for **boosting neuroplasticity**. Exercise boosts BDNF levels, which is especially helpful for growing the **hippocampus**, the part of your brain that turns short-term memories into long-term ones. Together, BDNF and GDNF make your brain more flexible and balanced, which is a big deal when you're recovering from a brain injury or struggling with memory and focus challenges. To reinforce this, a brand new study published in the International Journal of Behavioral Nutrition and Physical Activity found that those who did more moderate to vigorous physical activity than usual on a given day did much better in short-term memory tests the day after.[6]

Myth #2: "You Need to Wait a Long Time to Safely Exercise Again"

Research shows that starting aerobic exercise as early as **one-week after a mild or severe traumatic brain injury is safe and beneficial.** It can reduce symptoms, improve thinking skills, and speeding up recovery.[7] If you're feeling down, unmotivated, or weighed down, remember that exercise's benefits go beyond weight loss. **It's about shedding physical, mental, emotional, and even spiritual "baggage."** In just one workout, you can release neurochemicals like dopamine for pleasure, endorphins for pain relief, adrenaline for energy, serotonin for mood elevation, as well as GDNF and BDNF for more mental clarity and resilience. Boosting BDNF levels has been proven to strengthen neural connections in the hippocampus.[8] A brain region very important for memory consolidation. Together, BDNF and GDNF support cognitive flexibility and emotional regulation, which are especially vital in recovery from brain injuries.

We all have unlimited potential. **Our past doesn't define our future unless we allow it to.** By giving our body and mind the right stimulation through consistent exercise and mindful self-care, we allow our 37 trillion cells to thrive with renewed purpose and strength. No matter where you are in your recovery journey, you still need to get moving. Movement doesn't mean extreme workouts; it's about gentle, purposeful actions that get your blood flowing and your brain stimulated.

Myth 3: "Exercise Will Worsen Your Symptoms"

It's a common worry that moving your body after a brain injury will make things worse. Rightfully so! You might fear that exercise could exacerbate your headaches, dizziness, or fatigue. **But the truth is, while overdoing it can be harmful, the right type and dosage of movement actually speeds up your brain's healing process.** Studies show that gentle, controlled exercise improves **blood flow** and **oxygen** levels in the brain, which helps repair cells and boost mental clarity. [9] When you're careful to respect your limits and choose exercises suited to where you're at in recovery, movement can reduce symptoms rather than make them worse.

Take Action Today

Don't let injuries or outside circumstances prevent you from exercising. Don't let another day slip by while your brain and body remain stagnant. **I want you to imagine a recovery where you're not just healing but *thriving*.** You've read the science; you felt the urgency and heard my story, now it's time to create your own narrative. Commit to moving every day for the next 30 days. Just 10-20 minutes a day is all it takes to start creating a profound shift. This isn't about becoming an athlete overnight; it's about choosing, every day, to push a little closer towards the freedom that you deserve. Give your brain the oxygen, blood flow, and stimulation it craves. Break through the bs, toss out the excuses, and show yourself what's possible. Stand up and MOVE for the next month. Check off a mark every day on a calendar. Be accountable. Your brain, your future, and your life will thank you. Start today with Day 1. When your body moves your brain grooves!!!

THE THIRD STEP IS F FOR FUEL:

> *"Let Thy Medicine Be Thy Food, And Let Thy Food Be Thy Medicine"*
>
> — HIPPOCRATES

You have a Ferrari sitting in between your ears. It has over **86 billion cells** that are processing **11 million bits of information every second**, why fuel it with anything less than the best? Would you fuel a Ferrari with cheap gas? Of course not! So, why would you fuel the most important organ in your body with Starbucks, McDonald's and Jack Daniels?

Think about the coffee, processed, or alcoholic drinks you constantly reach for without thought. **Those are like pouring low-grade fuel into a high-performance car!** Instead, imagine filling up with premium fuel: fresh veggies, healthy fats, clean proteins.

Take it from my friend, TBI survivor, and thriver, Cavin Balaster, who learned this lesson the hard way. After he woke up from a coma, he ultimately realized the "nutrition" they were giving him was packed with high-fructose corn syrup. Yes seriously! Corn syrup. The cheap filler with ZERO nutritional value. And what's worse is it's sprayed with glyphosate, a toxic herbicide. Imagine that! Being fed pure sugar and chemicals while trying to overcome a horrific brain injury. Sadly, this isn't rare, and it is still standard protocol in hospitals around the world to this day. A word of caution. More than 80% of U.S. children and adults have traces of the herbicide glyphosate in their urine, according to data from the U.S. Centers for Disease Control and Prevention. [10]

You Are What You Eat

Every single thing you decide to put in your mouth either helps or hinders your brain's recovery. Just let that sink in for a minute. By choosing the right fuel, you're taking control of your healing process. Look, I know it's tempting to reach for what's convenient and tastes good in the moment but imagine how much different you are going to feel if you simply add the right fuel. Your brain cells need top-quality fuel to rebuild, repair, and get back to sharp, high-performance levels. It's not just about what you add to your diet; it's about what you choose to leave out. As Cavin says, brain recovery is like building a bridge. The nutrition is like the supplies of that bridge. Without supplies, you cannot build a bridge. That's why he wrote *How to Feed a Brain*, an amazing book about giving your brain what it actually needs to repair.

A general rule of thumb is if it is processed or manufactured you need to eliminate it from your diet. I honestly don't have a lot to say about nutrition because the science is rather straightforward. **Either the foods you eat will be helpful and fight against inflammation or they will be pro-inflammatory and contribute to it.** And believe me, if you want to improve your memory, you want the former, not the latter!

Now let's dive into how we can balance glucose levels through nutrition to maintain brain health.

Stable Energy, Sharper Memory: The Role of Glucose in Recovery

Glucose, or blood sugar, is our body's primary energy source, fueling everything from muscle contractions to brain function. Yet, maintaining balanced glucose levels is key to sustained energy, stable moods, and overall health. While our bodies are designed to handle occasional spikes and dips in blood sugar, chronic imbalance can lead to insulin resistance, type 2 diabetes, and metabolic health issues. Fortunately, nutrition plays a profound role in helping us regulate glucose levels naturally and effectively. Regulating glucose levels is key to taking pressure off your pancreas and kidneys.

Three Tips to Help Regulate Blood Glucose Levels

1. Prioritize High-Fiber Foods

Fiber slows down digestion, which helps to release glucose gradually into the bloodstream. Aim to include high-fiber foods in your meals, such as vegetables, certain fruits, whole grains, beans, and nuts. Fiber-rich foods not only help keep glucose levels steady but also support digestion and keep you feeling full longer.

2. Balance Carbohydrates with Protein and Fat

When you eat carbohydrates, pair them with a source of protein (like chicken, eggs, or beans) and healthy fats (like avocados, nuts, or olive oil). Protein and fats help slow the absorption of glucose, preventing spikes and keeping energy levels more stable throughout the day.

3. Watch Portion Sizes and Lower Sugar Consumption Levels

Eating smaller, balanced meals throughout the day can help prevent large blood sugar spikes. Try to avoid skipping meals, which can lead to glucose crashes, and aim to eat around the same times each day. Starting with a balanced breakfast can set the tone for stable blood sugar throughout the day.

DELICIOUS AND NUTRITIOUS BRAIN HEALTH FOODS:

You don't have to compromise. You can have both. And please! Don't tell me you don't have the money. You need to invest in healthy foods for your recovery. It's not a maybe, you must if you want to live better. Because health is the number one wealth.

Healthy Fats and Brain-Repairing Proteins

- **Wild-caught salmon:** High in omega-3s (DHA and EPA) for brain cell protection.
- **Grass-fed beef:** Contains higher omega-3 levels and Vitamin B12 for brain function.
- **Organic Chicken:** A clean protein source rich in B vitamins for energy and brain health.
- **Eggs:** High in choline, which boosts memory and neurotransmitter health.
- **Nuts and Seeds** (Almonds, Cashews, Brazil Nuts, Walnuts, and Pumpkin Seeds): High in magnesium, selenium, zinc, and omega-3s to stabilize mood and reduce inflammation.

Green Powerhouses

- **Spinach:** Packed with folate, magnesium, and vitamin K for cognitive function. Listen to what Popeye says!!!
- **Kale:** Another leafy green rich in antioxidants and anti-inflammatory compounds.
- **Broccoli:** Contains sulforaphane, a compound that aids in detoxifying the brain.
- **Brussels Sprouts:** Great source of Vitamin C and fiber to stabilize blood sugar for mental clarity.

Essential Herbs, Spices, and Superfoods

- **Turmeric:** Anti-inflammatory powerhouse that may boost memory and reduce brain fog.
- **Ginger:** Supports circulation and reduces oxidative stress in the brain.
- **Rosemary:** Boosts memory and focus.
- **Cacao (70%+ Dark Chocolate):** Contains flavonoids that enhance blood flow to the brain.

- **Green Tea:** Full of L-theanine, an amino acid that promotes relaxation without drowsiness.
- **Beets.** Full of Nitrates, which boost nitric oxide and helps increase blood flow to the brain, boosting mental clarity and focus. They also improve cognitive function and help protect against age-related decline.

Detoxifying and Sulfur-Rich Foods for Brain Health

- **Garlic:** Packed with sulfur compounds, garlic helps increase glutathione production, a powerful antioxidant that assists in detoxifying the brain and reducing inflammation. It's also known to boost circulation, delivering essential nutrients to brain cells.
- **Onions:** Rich in quercetin and sulfur, onions help protect brain cells from oxidative stress and support cognitive function.
- **Mushrooms** (especially **Lion's Mane** and **Reishi**): Mushrooms, particularly lion's mane, are known for their neuroprotective effects and ability to stimulate brain cell growth. Reishi supports immune health, which is essential for reducing systemic inflammation that impacts the brain.
- **Cruciferous Vegetables** (Broccoli, Cauliflower, Brussels Sprouts): These veggies are loaded with sulfur, supporting liver detoxification pathways and helping the body clear out toxins that can impact brain health.
- **Cabbage:** Contains sulfur and compounds called glucosinolates, which aid in detoxification and have been shown to protect against oxidative stress in the brain.
- **Asparagus:** High in antioxidants and glutathione, asparagus is a brain-protective vegetable that supports detoxification. (It also makes your pee smell funky)

Hydrating & Healing Beverages

- **Filtered Water:** Vital for hydration, which directly impacts brain performance.
- **Coconut Water:** Natural electrolytes to keep you hydrated and mentally sharp.
- **Bone Broth:** Full of amino acids like glycine, which support brain and gut health.

Foods to AVOID or ELIMINATE For Optimal Brain Health

Processed and Packaged Foods

- **Sugary Snacks:** Candy, pastries, and sugary cereals can lead to inflammation and spikes in blood sugar, negatively affecting mood and focus.
- **Fast Food:** High in unhealthy fats, sugars, and additives that can contribute to brain fog and inflammation.
- **Processed Meats:** Sausages, hot dogs, and deli meats are loaded with preservatives and unhealthy fats that can increase inflammation.

Refined Carbohydrates

- **White Bread and Pasta:** Made from refined flour, these can cause rapid blood sugar spikes, leading to energy crashes and cognitive issues.
- **White Rice:** Lacks fiber and nutrients compared to whole grains and can contribute to blood sugar imbalances.

High-sugar foods and Drinks

- **Soda and Energy Drinks:** Loaded with sugar and artificial ingredients that can harm brain health and lead to inflammation.

- **Artificial Sweeteners:** While low in calories, they can disrupt gut health and are linked to negative effects on mood and cognition.
- **High-Fructose Corn Syrup:** Common in many processed foods and sweeteners, this ingredient has been linked to inflammation and cognitive decline.

Unhealthy Fats

- **Trans Fats:** Often found in margarine, processed snacks, and baked goods; they can raise bad cholesterol and promote inflammation.
- **Excessive Saturated Fats:** Found in fatty cuts of meat and full-fat dairy, can negatively impact brain health and clog arteries if consumed in high amounts.

Foods High in Omega-6 Fatty Acids

- **Certain Vegetable Oils:** Corn oil, soybean oil, and canola oil are high in omega-6 fatty acids, which can promote inflammation when consumed in excess.

High-Sodium Foods

- **Canned Soups and Vegetables:** Often loaded with salt and preservatives, these can contribute to high blood pressure and negatively affect cognitive function.
- **Pickles and Processed Snacks:** Frequently high in sodium, which can lead to dehydration and cognitive issues.

Artificial Additives and Preservatives

- **Food Colorings and Dyes:** Commonly found in candies and processed foods, these have been linked to hyperactivity and behavioral issues in some individuals.

- **Preservatives:** Such as BHA and BHT, which can have negative effects on brain function.

Alcohol and Caffeine

- **Excessive Alcohol:** Can lead to cognitive decline and inflammation; moderation is ok, but elimination is even better. Alcohol are called "spirits" for a reason. It is a demon disguised as fun.
- **High-Caffeine Drinks:** While moderate caffeine may be fine, excessive amounts can lead to anxiety and disrupt sleep, which is crucial for brain recovery.

Potentially Allergenic Foods

- **Gluten:** For those with gluten sensitivity or celiac disease, gluten can cause inflammation and cognitive issues.

Dairy: Many modern-day dairy products and source can lead to digestive issues that can impact overall health and brain function.

Take Action! It's as Easy as A-B-C. 1-2-3

1. **Make Your Brainpower Grocery List:** Write down nutrients from the "Delicious and Nutritious Brainfoods" list from above. Prioritize whole, organic, fresh, and nutrient-rich foods.
2. **Shop and Stock Up:** Head to the store, pick up your items, and avoid the middle aisles that a full of processed foods. Fill your cart with foods that are proven to fuel your brain!
3. **Prep and Commit:** Prepare your food and cook them. Having brain-healthy options ready makes it easier to stay on track. (**Note:** Do not get discouraged if these foods are not available in your country or region. Do your best with the resources you have)

Bonus: Cut the **C.R.A.P.** — Carbonated Drinks, Refined Sugars, Artificial Colors, and Processed Products.

No Excuses!

In these early days of recovery, every bite counts. Your brain needs the right tools to rebuild itself, and the best tools are high-quality nutrients. Imagine the difference between stumbling through recovery or getting your memory and clarity back with each meal. This is your first step to nourishing your brain for recovery. You've got this!

THE FOURTH STEP IS O FOR OBSERVE:

> *"There's Only ONE Thing That Differentiates You, Me and Anyone Else from a Horse or a Pig.... And That Is Choice"*
>
> — JOHN ASSARAF

Imagine if every thought you had, every habit you practiced, could either trap you in your current reality or help unlock crystal-clear mental clarity. Self-observation is the key that opens the door to this transformation. By observing your thoughts, beliefs, emotions, actions, behaviors and habits without judgment, you build awareness, the first foundational step for lasting change.

Awareness gives us the ability to make new choices. Living life as a human being can be both a blessing and a curse. **We are our own best friend and worst enemy at times.** Because of the size of our neocortex (outer layer of the brain) we can make our thoughts as real as the outside world. In other words, we have an astounding ability to imagine. The great thing is that we can imagine ourselves doing incredible things, like speaking in front of a crowd of thousands, making love to our soulmate, or **hitting the game winning shot.** But, at the same time we also can get stressed out by thinking about 401k's, the stock market, or second mortgages. Society has programmed us to think that practicing imagination is a waste of time. I am going to prove to you that this is one of the greatest lies we have ever been told.

Now, I would love to refer to you incredible experiment to one of my favorite studies of all time, where scientists wanted to see how the brain changes through imagination.

Here's What They Did:

They gathered two groups: One group physically practiced a five-finger piano exercise. The other group only imagined doing the five-finger exercise but didn't touch the piano. Both repeated the exercise for 2 hours a day over a 5-day timespan. What they found is that both experienced similar cortical changes in the motor regions of the brain even though group 2 only imagined playing! In other words, the part of the brain that controls the movement of fingers got stronger and easier to activate in both groups. The big difference: The group that physically played the piano had bigger changes in their brain and learned the skill faster naturally, but the group that only imagined it still showed brain improvement, just not as much. [11]

Let that sink in couch Potatoes, this one is for you! This proves that visualization can prepare your brain for real-world action. Imagine the potential for memory improvement: by visualizing tasks, you can strengthen neural pathways, improve focus, and train your brain. **all without lifting a finger!**

But visualization is just the start. Strengthening your brain through **self-observation** is equally powerful. This process, known as **metacognition,** Metacognition allows you to **think about your thinking**, becoming aware of your thoughts and observing your own behaviors from a higher perspective. Practicing it allows blood flow to travel to our prefrontal cortex, which is responsible for higher-order thinking and decision-making. Begin to observe yourself from a bird's/third-eye perspective. In doing so, you will naturally strengthen your **memory,** attention, and focus! **Boomchakalaka!**

Powerful Ways to Practice Self-Observation

- **Breathing:** When you find yourself triggered from a life event, wanting to impulsively take an action, or even blurt out a random word, immediately pause and take a deep breath. This simple act disrupts the pattern, helping you regain focus and center yourself. Repeating this will increase your awareness in all aspects of life.
- **Journaling:** Write down your thoughts. Journaling allows you to spot patterns, triggers, and habits that may need to be changed, helping to improve self-awareness over time.
- **Imagine:** Imagine yourself as an observer, watching your life from above, like an eagle. This perspective helps you detach from emotions, see things more clearly, and shift your mindset. Repetition sharpens your ability to be present and aware.

Do You Have A "Happy Place"

Have you ever seen *Happy Gilmore*? There's a hysterical moment in the movie where Happy, the main character, is letting his emotions derail his focus. Shooter McGavin, his rival, is in his head, taunting him and throwing him off his game. Happy's frustration builds, his temper flares, and his performance tanks.

Then, his trainer and cabby, Chubbs, takes him to a mini-golf course to work on his concentration. But even there, Happy's anger keeps boiling over, and he struggles to stay composed. That's when Chubbs gives him some transformative advice:

"Think of a place that's perfect—*your own happy place. Go there, and all your anger will disappear.*" At first, Happy scoffs, but then he closes his eyes and starts to visualize. Mystical music plays, and Happy sees a bright, sunny day. In his mind's eye, his girlfriend is holding two frosty mugs of beer, smiling at him. Then, his grandmother hits the jackpot on a slot machine, coins cascading everywhere. Happy even sees a dwarf riding a tricycle! Whatever makes you Happy I guess! For Happy, this is his own private "happy place" that becomes a sanctuary, a mental retreat that shifts his focus, calms his emotions, and allows him to perform at his best.

In your recovery journey, **finding your own "happy place"** is just as crucial. Visualization and observation are powerful tools for rewiring your brain and refocusing your thoughts. By observing your inner state and shifting to a positive mental image, you can quiet the noise, manage frustration, and stay on track toward your goals. If Happy can retrain his brain to refocus, than so can you my friend.

Go to Your Happy Place in 3 Steps

1. **Pick It:** Think of a fun or calming place, like a beach, a candy store, or even somewhere with a dwarf on a tricycle! Whatever comes up for you that makes you happy!
2. **Picture It:** Close your eyes, take a deep breath, and imagine you're there. See it, hear it, feel it, smell it, touch it. Make it as real as possible in your mind.
3. **Use It:** When you're stressed, say, "Happy Place, here I come!" Close your eyes, breathe, and let the calm take over.

The journey to a better brain and a happier life starts now.

THE FIFTH STEP IS C FOR CONSISTENCY:

> *"Procrastination Is The Assassination Of Your Destination."*
>
> — EILEEN WILDER

Consistency, Consistency, Consistency. Let me say it one more time because it's the backbone of everything. **CONSISTENCY!** Let me make this crystal clear. If you want to truly get your life back--to remember names, stay sharp in conversations, and feel clear-headed again, consistency is the key to unlocking those outcomes. Consistency is how you take procrastination by the neck and knock it out cold like a **Mike Tyson super punch.** Ultimately, in recovery, you're not just working to repair your brain, you're rebuilding your freedom and future. If you want your brain to function like it's supposed to, you need to make consistency your new religion! It's not negotiable. You don't just wake up one day and have everything fixed after a brain injury.

You've had a brain injury, and that means parts of your brain, especially the areas responsible for memory, have been damaged. But here's the good news: your brain can rebuild itself. That's called neuroplasticity. And the secret to unlocking it? You guessed it. Consistency! Do you want your brain to heal? Then you better show up for it every damn day.

Look at your brain injury like a damaged house after it got hit by a hurricane. You don't fix it by throwing down a little patchwork here and there or working on a bit of it once a week. No, you rebuild that house brick by brick, layer by layer, day in and day out. Think of every consistent day as adding another brick to the foundation of your recovery. Some days you lay a single brick; other days you might finish a whole wall. But every single day of works counts to rebuild your brain to become stronger and more resilient than before. That's how you heal your brain after an injury. Consistent effort rewires your neural pathways, making your memory stronger, sharper, and more resilient.

Get obsessed with consistency. Consistency is perhaps the most important concept in this entire book that you need to embody. **It is one of the most immovable forces in the entire universe.** Everyone is consistent in some way, believe it or not. Most people are great complainers, blamers, shamers, and finger-pointers. **Don't be like most people!**

Your brain craves routine for its memory. When you put in the work, day after day, your brain starts adapting. You're training it to rebuild itself. You want a better memory? You want to eliminate brain fog? Consistency is how you do it. Look how the sun consistently, day after day, comes up and keeps burning. Look at nature. The sun doesn't just rise every other day, does it? It shows up every single day, without fail, burning with the same intensity, whether anyone's watching or not. That's what you need to be. Unstoppable. Immovable. Like gravity itself. Consistency is the most powerful force in the universe, and when you harness it, nothing can stop you.

There are two important steps in this process.

The first requirement. You must believe in the power of consistency.

The second requirement. You must be consistent by consistently taking action!

Let's make this very, very clear:

- If you don't believe in the power of consistency and you're not consistent, you will feel down and your memory will never be as sharp as it could be.
- If you don't believe in the power of consistency, but are consistent, you'll end up frustrated and disappointed in your results.

- If you believe in the power of consistency, but aren't consistent, your memory will stay weak and you'll feel like you're always falling short.
- Finally! If you believe in the power of consistency and you stay consistent, your memory will become razor sharp, and you'll feel more confident and capable every day!

Action Step

Start small. I'm not asking you to spend 10 hours every day working on your recovery. That's not realistic. But what is realistic—and incredibly effective—is just 5 measly minutes a day! If you dedicate just 5 minutes a day to specific memory exercises or any recovery activity you will see the results. Let's do the math together: 5 times 365= 1,825 minutes. Divide that by 60 for the number of minutes in an hour, that adds up to over 30 hours in a year!

That's more than an entire day's worth of focused work on your brain! Consistency, Consistently Compounds!

THE SIXTH STEP IS U FOR UNDERSTAND:

> *"Understand That There Is A Universe Within You."*
>
> — UNKNOWN

Understanding the fundamental workings of the brain like how it functions and how it adapts, is arguably the most crucial element of your early recovery journey.

When you understand the **WHAT** and **WHY** of any subject, the **HOW becomes much easier.** This principle is especially important to the realm of brain health. My primary goal with the patients I work with is to equip them with a foundational understanding of how the brain functions—and how it doesn't—so they can apply this knowledge to their lives. After all, the word **'Doctor' comes from the Latin 'docere,' which means 'to teach.'** Teaching isn't just part of my role, it's at the very heart of what it means to be a doctor. With a solid grasp of the basics, you become less vulnerable to the influences of so-called experts who "know what's best for you." We live in a time when knowledge and information are readily accessible to anyone who seeks it. However, acquiring knowledge alone is not enough for true empowerment. Mastering the basics repeatedly is the key to any endeavor. In this chapter, my aim is to provide you with a solid foundation in understanding how the brain works. As we discussed earlier, the brain is the most important organ in the human body. Ever wondered what parts of your brain make you who you are? Let's dive into the key regions that define your thoughts, emotions, and actions.

10 Essential Brain Regions That Shape Who You Are

Just like each part of our body has its own functions, different parts of the brain have their own jobs too. Neuroscientists have made amazing strides in understanding these connections, showing us that damage to a specific brain area can lead to challenges linked to it's function. **What's astonishing is we learned more about the brain in the last 10 years, than the last 10,000!** Isn't it fascinating how interconnected our bodies and minds are? To better understand these crucial regions, let's explore the functions and potential impacts of damage to each one, beginning with the "frontal lobe.

The Frontal Lobe (located at the front of the brain): The frontal lobe is responsible for decision-making, problem-solving, emotional regulation, personality, attention, planning, speech, movement, impulse control, short-term memory, thinking in terms of past and future, and more.

Damage to the frontal lobe can lead to issues with impulsiveness, planning, mood swings, concentration, memory issues, and more...

The Parietal Lobe (located at upper back part of your brain, behind the top of your head)

The parietal lobe is responsible for the perception of pain, touch, temperature, spatial awareness, sequencing, and mathematics.

Damage can result in difficulties with sensory perception, coordination, and navigating environments. It can result in a condition known as neglect, where you can become unaware of one side of their body or their surroundings.

The Temporal Lobe (located next to the ears): The temporal lobe is responsible for hearing, emotions, auditory processing, comprehension, memory retrieval, auditory-formed memories, and general memory.

Damage to the temporal lobe can cause problems with memory formation, language processing, and processing sounds. People may also experience difficulties in recognizing familiar faces or objects, known as prosopagnosia.

Occipital Lobe (located at the back of the brain): The occipital lobe is responsible for the formation of visual memories and visual processing.

Damage can lead to issues with visual perception, color recognition, and reading.

People may also experience visual field deficits, where they lose sight in certain areas of their visual field.

Brainstem: The brainstem is responsible for controlling vital functions such as heart rate, breathing, and blood pressure.

Damage can cause problems with autonomic functions (such as irregular heartbeats or breathing patterns), decreased alertness, impaired reflex responses, and can even be life-threatening.

Cerebellum (located at the back of the brain, underneath the occipital lobe): The cerebellum or "mini brain" is responsible for accuracy, balance, coordination (often referred to as the A, B, C's of motor skills), and muscle tone regulation. It fine-tunes movements and helps maintain posture.

Damage can result in difficulties with motor control, balance, coordination, and fine motor skills. People may experience tremors, dizziness, and challenges with tasks requiring precise movements.

Hippocampus (located within the temporal lobe): The hippocampus is responsible for memory formation, particularly in converting short-term memories into long-term ones, as well as spatial navigation. It plays a significant role in learning and contextual memory.

Damage can lead to difficulties with long-term memory, learning new information, and retrieving past memories. People may suffer from **anterograde amnesia**, making it hard to form new memories after an injury.

Thalamus (located at the top of the brain stem): The thalamus is responsible for filtering brain activity. This includes deleting, distorting, and generalizing information. Often referred to as the "thalamic gate," it relays sensory and motor signals to the cerebral cortex.

Damage can lead to problems with sensory processing, altered states of consciousness, and sleep regulation issues, potentially resulting in insomnia or hypersomnia.

Amygdala (located deep within the temporal lobes): The amygdala is responsible for emotion regulation, fear processing, and the formation of emotional memories. It plays a critical role in assessing threats and triggering appropriate emotional responses.

Damage can result in issues with emotional responses (such as difficulty identifying or expressing emotions) and changes in social behavior, making it hard to relate to others in social contexts.

PARIETAL LOBE

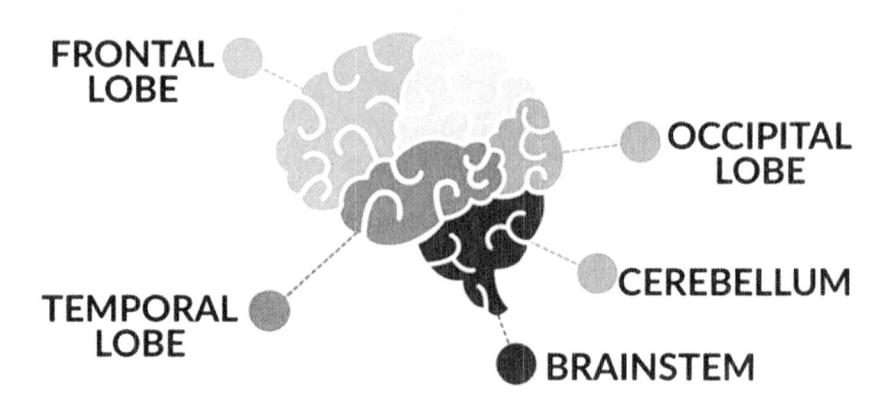

FRONTAL LOBE

OCCIPITAL LOBE

TEMPORAL LOBE

CEREBELLUM

BRAINSTEM

Alex Honnold's Fearless Brain: What Makes Him Different?

Deep in the towering granite walls of Yosemite National Park, Alex Honnold prepared for the climb that would make him famous: El Capitan, without ropes. For most people, even thinking about this would make their **amygdala**—the part of the brain that controls fear—go into overdrive. Their palms would sweat, their heart would race, and their whole body would feel panicked at the idea of being so high up with no safety ropes.

But Alex was different. **Neuroscientists studied Alex's brain** because they were amazed by how little fear he felt. Scans of his amygdala showed something incredible: it was much quieter than in most people. **While other people's amygdala's would react strongly to danger, Alex's stayed calm.** This unusual feature of his brain allowed him to stay focused and plan carefully instead of being overwhelmed by fear. Alex Honnold's story shows how **different brains can work in very unique ways.** While one person might see something as impossible, someone like Alex might see it as a challenge they can figure out. It's a reminder that differences in our brains don't just shape who we are but also how we deal with the world around us.

Understanding Your Brain: The First Step in Your Journey

This chapter has introduced you to some important areas of the brain, but this is just the beginning. To truly **UNDERSTAND** what's going on inside your own brain and address the root causes of memory loss or other brain health issues, you'll need to go over this information again and again. Think of it like training a muscle, each repetition strengthens the neural connections in your brain, making this knowledge stick and helping you apply it to real life.

Every new bit of information you absorb about your brain is another step toward recovery. It's a journey that requires patience, repetition, and commitment. But remember, the more you understand your brain, the more control you gain over your recovery process. Keep learning, and with time, you'll not only understand your brain better, you'll start to feel stronger, more confident, and more in charge of your healing path.

THE SEVENTH STEP IS S FOR SUPPLEMENTATION:

Alright, let's talk about supplementation. After a **concussion**, your brain gets knocked out of balance, shifting into "**survival mode.**" This can lead to **deficiencies** in key neurotransmitters like serotonin, dopamine, and GABA—chemicals that play a big role in mood, focus, and calmness. With these imbalances, the nervous system needs extra support to repair and recover.

This is where **supplementation comes in handy.** By providing essential vitamins, minerals, and nutrients, supplements can fill in the gaps needed for the brain to rebuild and rebalance. Omega-3s, magnesium, and B vitamins, for instance, support brain health and help restore neurotransmitter levels, while antioxidants like curcumin reduce brain inflammation that can worsen imbalances.

Remember, supplements are just one part of the recovery plan. Combined with good nutrition, rest, brain exercises, and stress management, they give your brain the best chance to heal fully and get back on track.

Below is a list I call the **RESCUE FORMULA**, featuring ten of my favorite supplements to support concussion recovery. These have proven to reduce symptoms, support **memory,** cognitive function, and overall brain health for concussion survivors.

1. CREATINE (MONOHYDRATE) (Not only for gym bros...)

Once thought to be only for boosting muscle recovery and performance, new data shows that it improves memory, provides neuroprotection, lowers blood sugar, strengthens cognitive functioning, and boosts brain energy metabolism (ATP) levels. [10] [11]

2. LION'S MANE

It's one of the most promising natural compounds for neurogenesis and neuroprotection. Research shows it enhances the production of nerve growth factor (NGF), which is essential for the maintenance, growth, and survival of neurons. This amazing mushroom can improve memory, focus, and cognitive function by promoting brain cell regeneration, potentially reversing damage from aging or injury. Its effects on neuroplasticity—the brain's ability to adapt and form new connections, make it invaluable for overall brain health and recovery from neurological trauma. [12]

3. OMEGA 3-FATTY ACIDS (FISH OIL)

Omega-3 fatty acids, particularly DHA (docosahexaenoic acid) and EPA (eicosatetraenoic acid) are vital for brain cell repair and reducing brain inflammation. These essential fatty acids are a cornerstone for cognitive health because they maintain the fluidity of cell membranes and support the growth of synapses, which are critical for learning and memory. Omega-3s also play a huge role in reducing the risk of neurodegenerative diseases like Alzheimer's, improving mood regulation, and lowering anxiety and depression levels. [13] (This isn't to be confused with regular, fatty asses, like if you went to the local Tuscaloosa Walmart in Alabama. I'm joking guys don't get too offended)

4. TURMERIC AND CURCUMIN

Curcumin, the active compound in turmeric, is a powerful anti-inflammatory and antioxidant that crosses the blood-brain barrier. It helps reduce oxidative stress and chronic inflammation, which are linked to cognitive decline and neurodegenerative diseases such as Alzheimer's and Parkinson's. Curcumin also stimulates BDNF (Brain-Derived Neurotrophic Factor), which is critical for neurogenesis and maintaining cognitive health. Its neuroprotective properties make it a valuable supplement for improving memory, attention, and mood. (Pro-tip: Take with black pepper to improve bioavailability) [14]

5. MAGNESIUM

Magnesium is one of the most important minerals in your entire body. Did you know that magnesium fuels over 700 biochemical reactions? It plays a central and critical role in maintaining healthy brain function. It supports synaptic plasticity and regulates neurotransmitter activity. Magnesium also has calming effects on the nervous system by lowering cortisol levels, and upregulating the release of GABA, a neurotransmitter that helps reduce stress and anxiety. Low magnesium levels are linked to a higher risk of cognitive disorders and mood imbalances, making it an essential nutrient for brain health. Sadly, around 50% of Americans are not getting the proper amount of magnesium. [15] Don't be like most people. Add more magnesium into your diet and through supplementation.

6. GINKGO BILOBA

Ginkgo Biloba is one of the most well-researched herbs for improving cognitive function. It is well known for its ability to enhance blood flow to the brain; ginkgo is proven to enhance memory, focus, and mental sharpness. Ginkgo's role is to support vascular health and promote neuroprotection through its antioxidant effects. Studies show that it can be particularly useful in preventing age-related cognitive decline and may also help in conditions like anxiety and depression, which are often linked to cognitive deficits. Its use is particularly important following a concussion when the brain's blood flow can be compromised, leading to cognitive dysfunctions like memory loss. By improving oxygen delivery and reducing oxidative damage, ginkgo helps support the brain's natural repair processes. It has also been shown to enhance synaptic plasticity, which aids in memory recovery and helps speed up cognitive rehabilitation after a brain. [16]

7. B-COMPLEX.

B vitamins are essential for energy production, brain cell function, and neurotransmitter synthesis. These vitamins play a critical role in neurorehabilitation after a concussion. This group of eight essential vitamins—B1 (thiamine), B2 (riboflavin), B3 (niacin), B5 (pantothenic acid), B6 (pyridoxine), B7 (biotin), B9 (folate), and B12 (cobalamin)—supports brain function at multiple levels, especially during recovery. They support the production of serotonin, dopamine, and other key neurotransmitters affected by a concussion. [17]

8. VITAMIN D and VITAMIN K2

Vitamin D and K2 are extremely important for improving memory, especially after a brain injury. Vitamin D helps regulate chemicals in the brain, like serotonin and dopamine, which support mood and thinking. It also helps create new brain cells, which is important for learning and remembering things. Vitamin K2 works with Vitamin D to make sure calcium goes to the bones and teeth instead of building up in the brain. This helps keep blood flowing to the brain, providing the oxygen and nutrients it needs to work well. Together, these vitamins support better memory and are essential for recovery after a concussion. Most people are vitamin D deficient, often due to a lack of sunlight exposure, especially during the winter months. Factors like indoor lifestyles, use of sunscreen, and dark skin can also contribute to low levels. Dietary sources are limited, making supplementation essential for many to achieve optimal health.

9. L-THEANINE

Concussions can lead to chronic stress, poor focus, and memory deficits due to the dysregulation of neurotransmitters. L-theanine helps by promoting a state of calm alertness, reducing stress while enhancing alpha brainwave activity, which is associated with improved memory and attention. By balancing levels of GABA and dopamine, L-Theanine reduces post-injury anxiety and supports better memory retention, allowing the brain to focus on recovery and repair.

10. ELECTROLYTES

Essential for maintaining the balance of fluids and supporting proper brain function, especially following a concussion. Think of them like little workers your brain needs to stay sharp and balanced. Electrolytes include things like sodium (salt), potassium, calcium, chloride, and phosphate. Each one has a special job to help you feel better after a brain injury.

Sodium and Potassium help maintain proper fluid balance within cells, and are important for the generation of electrical impulses, which is vital for brain function.

Calcium is necessary for neurotransmitter release and plays a role in neuroplasticity, which is important for cognitive recovery after brain injuries.

Chloride: Often paired with sodium to help maintain fluid balance, it plays an important role in the proper functioning of cells, tissues, and organs. It helps regulate the body's pH level and supports electrolyte balance, which is crucial for nerve function after a concussion. Chloride helps maintain hydration, which is important for overall recovery.

Phosphate: This electrolyte is essential for energy production and maintaining the integrity of cell membranes. It works closely with calcium in the bones and is involved in processes that support brain cell repair and energy metabolism. Phosphate levels can be affected by a concussion, which can impair brain function and recovery.

Ensuring proper intake of these electrolytes, especially after a brain injury helps to support brain cell function and enhances recovery.

GUT HEALTH MATTERS

Now, let me ask you a very important question. **What good does eating all the right foods and spending thousands of dollars on supplementation matter if you end up pooping it all out?** If you answered with the words **NONE** or **ZERO,** then you Sir or Madam are 100% correct! Sorry, not sorry to be vulgar, but I don't want you to literally SH*T out all your hard-earned money! This was a hard realization for me, too, at the time when I was dealing with an unhealthy leaky gut.

Ask yourself these questions...

- Am I bloated, gassy, feeling gut pain, or diarrhea?
- Am I regular?
- Can I digest most healthy, whole, and organic foods properly?
- Or Do I Have Tons of Food Allergies?

If the answer is yes to one or more of the above, then we need to help you address your digestive health.

Did you know that 90% of the serotonin in your body is produced in your gut? [18]

There are over 100 million neurons in your microbiome, and new research shows that gut health is closely connected to our memory and cognitive function. And that connection is powerful. A healthy gut is not only for physical well-being but also for mental clarity and emotional balance. Let's focus on healing your gut so you can truly benefit from the food you eat and the supplements you take. Now, I can't spend too much time in this book on the gut-brain axis because that's not what it's about. Perhaps in another book. But just know that it is extremely important.

Basics Steps for Gut-Health Care

1. Eat pre-biotic fermented foods like kimchi or sauerkraut.
2. Lower Stress Levels and prioritize sleep.
3. Eat healthy, whole, and organic foods.
4. Supplement with HCL (Hydrochloric acid) to raise the acidity of the stomach.
5. Take Pro-biotics.

Ready for a brain break? Scan this code for 15 free memory exercises and early access to exclusive offers by going to www.dr-bro.com/vipbrairescue or scanning the QR code below

CHAPTER FIVE: THE SECOND PILLAR: E IS FOR E.N.G.A.G.E

After a brain injury, re-engaging your brain's natural ability to store and recall information is crucial. The **"Engage"** phase is all about waking up your brain's memory centers through active participation, deliberate exercises, and consistent mental engagement. By focusing on stimulating your brain, you can accelerate memory recovery and strengthen your cognitive abilities. For this recovery process to work, you must ENGAGE in daily non-negotiable recovery habits. I mean habits that you participate in 5-7 days a week for 10-15 minutes at a time, even on days when you don't feel like doing them.

THE FIRST STEP IS E FOR EXPERIENCE:

> *"Experience Is The Teacher Of All Things."*
>
> — JULIUS CAESAR

Our brains are amazing and always changing, thanks to a principle called **experience-dependent plasticity**. This means our brains aren't fixed like a statue, but flexible and can reshape themselves based on what we go through in life. By experiencing new things, our brains create new connections, and this ability lasts throughout our entire lives. Personally, I like to think of it as action-dependent plasticity, focusing on how what we do shapes our brains.

Why? Because most of our life experiences, are shaped directly by the actions we take and the habits we form. Humans are creatures of habit for a good reason. Consider this: every micro decision you make, every habit you cultivate, every challenge you confront, these are not only moments in time. They are powerful catalysts for creating change that lasts.

Improving Your Memory From Your Actions

Imagine being able to physically strengthen your memory just by what you do every day. That's exactly what happened in a fascinating study involving London taxi drivers. These drivers are required to memorize thousands of streets and landmarks across the city. Researchers found that the more years of driving and navigation experience the taxi drivers had, the larger a part of their brain called the hippocampus became. The hippocampus is crucial for **long-term memory** and **spatial navigation**, and this study showed that it grew bigger the more the drivers practiced. [19]

Understanding that our actions can shape our brains gives us more agency over our own brain health. We aren't just passive observers; we actively shape our lives through our choices. By focusing on positive actions, like learning new skills, being mindful, or building good relationships, we can use the power of our brains to become stronger and more resilient.

So, think about it: what actions are you taking today that will help create better experiences for your future?

Take Action to Create More Experiences

Here's a tangible action for you: Each day, set aside a specific time, perhaps right after breakfast or before bed, to practice a simple memory exercise. Start by choosing a list of five words (like apple, chair, ocean, book, and sun) and spend 10 minutes memorizing them. Once you feel comfortable, try to recall the words without looking. Each time you succeed, challenge yourself by adding more words or even making sentences with them. This daily practice not only strengthens your memory but also reinforces the connections in your brain.

Listen, the path to recovery is not always easy, but with persistence, faith and dedication, you can achieve lasting change. You have the ability to transform your experiences into opportunities for growth, and every effort you make will contribute to your healing journey. So, rise up, take action, and engage fully in your recovery. Your future self will thank you!

THE SECOND STEP IS N FOR NITRIC OXIDE: (THE UNSUNG HERO FOR BRAIN AND BODY RECOVERY)

Do you know there's **ONE game-changing molecule** for your health that you can boost naturally that traditional medicine doesn't want you to know about?

Meet Nitric Oxide (NO) – your secret weapon that can supercharge your recovery and enhance your memory. Boost it, and you'll unlock better blood flow to your brain, skyrocket your energy, and accelerate your healing process like never before.

So, what is NO? It's a colorless gas and one of the key players in nitrogen. As a vasodilator, it opens up your blood vessels, allowing more oxygen and nutrients to flow directly to your brain.

At the end of the day, recovery is simply a game of blood flow and oxygen.

What Nitric Oxide Does for Your Brain:

- **Vasodilator:** It relaxes and widens your blood vessels, ramping up blood flow where it matters most…your brain. More blood flow means more nutrients and oxygen for enhanced memory recovery.
- **Boosts Mitochondrial Biogenesis:** This means it helps your body create more mitochondria, the energy powerhouses of your cells. More mitochondria lead to more energy, which is crucial when your brain is healing.
- **Supercharges Mitochondrial Function:** With NO in action, those mitochondria not only multiply but work more efficiently, giving you more energy with less oxygen. This means sharper focus and quicker recovery from cognitive fatigue.

Let me let you in on a secret fellas, ladies, whoever. Did you know the reason Viagra works so well is because of Nitric Oxide? Yup because it improves blood flow to you know where. Stronger blood flow=stronger erection. But you don't need to take Viagra you just need to practice breathing better. You can thank me later.

The Science Of Nasal Breathing

Bear with me. I'm going to get a little geeky with you. **When you breathe in through your nose, several powerful physiological processes** kick into gear that helps **boost Nitric Oxide.** Your **nasal cavity** is lined with specialized cells that produce nitric oxide. When you inhale through your nose, you draw air directly into these cells, allowing the NO to mix with the incoming air. This leads to a direct increase in the amount of nitric oxide entering your bloodstream. Nose breathing is incredible for health. To boost your nitric oxide (NO) levels, start by practicing deep nasal breathing to replace shallow, anxious breaths; just a few minutes every hour can help increase energy levels. You can also incorporate these simple habits below into your daily routine.

5 Proven Ways Of Boosting No Levels

NO production helps calm your nervous system.

- **Exercise regularly**, as physical activity stimulates your body to produce more nitric oxide, even light stretching, or brisk walking can make a difference.
- **Fuel up with greens** like spinach, kale, and arugula, which are rich in nitrates that your body converts into NO, promoting better circulation and memory.
- **Spend time outdoors** in the sunlight to stimulate NO production through UV light exposure, which also enhances energy levels.
- **Stay hydrated** by drinking plenty of water, as it supports overall bodily functions and aids in NO production.
- **Practicing** deep, continuous, and intense **nasal breathing** stimulates NO levels.

5 HIDDEN "NORMAL" THINGS THAT SABOTAGE NO LEVELS

Certain everyday habits could be sabotaging your nitric oxide levels without you realizing it. For instance.

- **Mouthwash** may freshen your breath, but it also destroys the good bacteria needed to convert dietary nitrates into NO.
- **Fluoride toothpaste** can inhibit the body's ability to produce NO.
- If you frequently take **antacids**, be aware that they might hinder your stomach's NO production by reducing essential stomach acid.
- **Processed foods** also do little for your NO levels, so stick to nutrient-rich, whole foods to optimize your health.

- A **lack of sleep** sabotages NO levels.

Action Step: BOOST Your Nitric Oxide Levels Fast!

Instructions: For 2 Minutes, Breathe in Through Your Nose

1. Find a comfortable position. Sit or stand in a relaxed posture.
2. Close your mouth and take a long, slow, deep and steady breath through your nose.
   - (Pro-Tip INHALE AS LONG AND DEEPLY AS HUMANLY POSSIBLE)
3. Hold for a second, then exhale vigorously through your mouth.
4. Repeat this for 2 minutes.

THE THIRD STEP IS G FOR GRATITUDE:

> *"Gratitude Makes Sense Of Our Past, Brings Peace For Today, And Creates A Vision For Tomorrow."*
>
> — MELODY BEATTIE

In my early to mid-20s, I don't remember ever using the word gratitude.

Gratitude is an absolute must in your recovery. **I truly believed that someone couldn't be happy without drugs, alcohol, money, or sex.** Something on the outside of ourselves.

But the truth is that it is a feeling that is cultivated from within. Gratitude is one of the best antidotes to stress and frustrations you will experience in your memory recovery journey.

So, after my injury, I was removed from everything in my life.

I had to re-learn how to think, act, speak and remember. So, I was forced to look within. It is a feeling that we get when we look at what we currently have as enough.

Gratitude has been shown to positively affect many aspects of mental and emotional health, including memory. A study published in *Frontiers in Psychology* in 2017 examined the impact of gratitude journaling on memory formation and recall. [20] Participants who practiced gratitude by writing down things they were thankful for had improved recall of both positive and neutral events in their lives. Gratitude enhances the encoding of positive events into memory and improves recall, partly because it reduces stress, a factor that impairs memory.

It is also closely lined to the ventromedial prefrontal cortex, which is an area tied to decision-making, emotional regulation, and empathy. [21] Practicing gratitude will strengthen all these abilities. Gratitude starts from within and is a skill that you get better at over time with practice. I promise you that you can be grateful even on your worst days. Gratitude helps silence that dark inner voice. That **monkey mind** that distracts and **lies to you.** You know that voice that says: **"You're not good enough" "You're not worth it." "You're not going to make it." "Who do you think you are to be doing this or that?"** And so many other lies…Don't listen to it. Instead, connect to your higher self by practicing gratitude.

Let me be completely honest with you, friend. I am not proud of this at all. In the past, I had to go to jail for multiple DUIs. Only a few days of drinking led to the arrest. Prior to my relapse, I had 3 years of sobriety, and the only thing that kept me going in the right direction was **gratitude** for the simple things. Like the fact I was alive, that I had support from my family, I had food, and I was healthy. Was it easy? Hell No! I sure had plenty of negative moments along the way, but it allowed me to become a better person than I was before jail. It was absolutely terrifying on days when I thought I would have everything taken from me. The jailers were threatening to lock us away in segregation for weeks if we tested positive for Covid-19. We're talking a 23 ½ hour lock-down in a 4 by 6 cell. No, BS! In fact, some of my fellow inmates in my pod tested positive and were taken to segregation for 2 weeks at a time. But, even with the immense fear of testing positive weighing over my head, I told myself that even if that happens, I can still find gratitude in that cell that will help me grow into a better person. **Gratitude was the strength that helped me move forward.** Luckily, it didn't happen to me, but I am just telling you, that you have more strength within you than you would ever imagine Warrior!

Action Step: Start Small and Build Yourself Up with Gratitude

Step 1: At the beginning or end of each day think about three things that you are grateful for.

Step 2: Slow down your breathing and close your eyes.

Step 3: Feel into the emotion of gratitude, no matter how strong or how weak it feels.

I promise you that even if you can feel the tiniest bit of gratitude, no matter how small, you can build up and grow the emotion over time. You got this Warrior!

THE FOURTH STEP IS A FOR ANTERIOR CINGULATE CORTEX: (YOUR WARRIOR BRAIN)

> *"The Moment You Want To Give Up Is The Exact Moment you need to keep going. That's where your strength lies. That's where change happens"*
>
> — UNKNOWN

If you want to forge your path to recovery and unleash the full power of your brain, you need to tap into **your anterior cingulate cortex (ACC), the epicenter of your warrior spirit.** This part of your brain is where resilience is born, where you build the courage to push through, and where transformation becomes inevitable. A crucial element of brain recovery isn't just about what we actively pursue; it's also about what we **resist doing.** Our brains are "**use it or lose it**" organs, just like the rest of our bodies. Think about it this way: when you hit the gym consistently, your muscles grow and get stronger. But if you neglect that discipline, your hard-earned gains start to fade away. The same principles apply to your brain cells. They thrive on the activities you engage in, but they can also shrink when you stop doing that activity. This is incredibly important for you to understand! **The brain ALWAYS takes the path of least resistance,** but it is your job to create healthy patterns that you do so often that they become automatic. In other words, they become the path of least resistance for your brain!

Now, let's talk more about the anterior cingulate cortex. This part of your brain is crucial in this transformative journey. Recent studies show that when people tackle activities they initially resist, their ACC actually gets bigger. [22]

Think about that! In people who struggle with obesity, this brain region tends to be smaller. But in athletes and people who see themselves as overcoming challenges, the ACC grows significantly. To do this in the right way, **YOU NEED to replace old bad habits with good ones.** It's not enough to create healthy habits. You also MUST eliminate old behaviors for a better life.

The ACC is your Warrior brain! But it only becomes that Warrior if you see yourself as a Warrior! So, how do you foster that Warrior mindset daily? It's simple: by creating non-negotiable habits and cultivating non-negotiable energy. **Every time you choose to engage in an activity that builds you up or resist an urge that pulls you down, you are directly strengthening your ACC.**

But it doesn't stop there! You're also fortifying your frontal lobe, hippocampus, and other vital brain regions connected to memory. When you push through the resistance, whether it's staying focused on a task, solving a tough problem, or avoiding distractions, you are paving the way for stronger connections and pathways in your brain.

So, here's the challenge, every time you face an obstacle, whether it's a fleeting urge to give up or the fatigue that tells you to quit, dig deep and engage your warrior spirit. Remember, your brain is a powerhouse of resilience. Embrace the struggle! Celebrate every small victory! The harder you work against the resistance, the more powerful your mind becomes.

Take Action Now! Write down one non-negotiable habit you will commit to every day for the next week. Make it something that challenges you, something that requires you to show up for yourself, even when you don't want to. It could be a workout, a meditation session, or even studying something new.

Don't back down! Every time you **conquer** that challenge, you're not just building a habit; you're building a stronger, more resilient warrior inside you. Let's turn that ACC into a fortress and watch your mind sharpen like a sword. Are you a Warrior who takes action, or a Worrier who doesn't? It's time to step up and show the world who you are!

THE FIFTH STEP IS G FOR GAMIFY IT:

When it comes to rebuilding your **memory**, think of the word "**gamify**." I mean this is about making your daily activities as ENGAGING and **FUN** as you possibly can. Rebuilding your memory isn't about going back to who you used to be. It's about leveling up and becoming something greater. Picture your recovery journey like a **video game**, where you're the hero navigating through levels, unlocking new skills, and picking up power-ups along the way.

The only difference is, **instead of slaying dragons, you're taking on scattered thoughts, brain fog, and lapses in memory after a brain injury.** It might feel like your brain has betrayed you, leaving you with mental fatigue and a scattered mind. But here's the truth: your memory isn't gone; it just needs a new path forward. Neuroplasticity is the amigo on your side. Your job is to make this rewiring fun and engaging, so fun that you can't wait to do it. This is where "gamifying" your recovery comes into play. Remember, the more fun we make so-called "mundane or boring" activities, the quicker we can reinforce things and make them automatic.

Turn Stats into Milestones. Track Your Progress Like a Game

In life, you need to track where you are now to know where you are going. Think of tracking your weight on a scale. Its important because it shows you how to adjust! To be honest, in the early stages of my practice, I used to think that consistently tracking health statistics was doing a disservice to my patients. But the issue I run into time and time again is that people have no idea where they are going or what to improve until they can prove to themselves, that they are on the right track and getting better.

Let's start with three of my currently favorite wearables that I love using with my patients to measure we they are going and to gamify things.

- **HeartMath Inner Balance:** Tracks Heart Rate, HRV, Mood and Heart Coherence.
- **Oura Ring:** Tracks Total Sleep, REM Sleep, Deep Sleep, and Efficiency.
- **Apple Watch:** Checks Vo2 Max, Exercise time, and Calories Burnt.

Setting weekly and monthly goals can be very helpful, whether they are quantitative and measurable or qualitative and subjective. When you hit it, reward yourself. Maybe it's a break, a favorite treat, or just a moment to soak in the progress. Make it a ritual to celebrate every win, no matter how small.

The Science of Play: Why Making It Fun Works

This isn't just about having fun; it's about unlocking the full potential of your brain. Neuroscience shows us that engaging in playful, enjoyable activities releases dopamine, the brain's "feel-good" chemical. **Dopamine doesn't just boost your mood; it also primes your brain for learning and memory formation.** When you turn mind gym exercises into a game, whether it's challenging yourself to remember a list of items in record time or trying to beat your last meditation score, you're not just going through the motions. You're training your brain to adapt and grow.

In the book *Play* by Dr. Stuart Brown, he explains that play is not a luxury but a necessity. [23] It's through play that we develop new pathways in the brain, exactly what you need to strengthen memory after a concussion. So, when you turn each day's recovery activities into a game, you're not just making things more enjoyable, you're accelerating your brain's ability to heal. I mean that is exactly what animals do, because there is a clear evolutionary advantage to it. It's a way to test our God-given abilities before being placed into a more serious situation. I mean just look at your dog during the day. If you don't have a dog, I strongly recommend that you do get one, one day. He/She will play around, growl and run around. This gets the dog moving and more prepared if a serious situation does come along.

THE SIXTH STEP IS E FOR ENERGY:

> *"If You Want To Know The Secrets Of The Universe, Think In Terms Of Energy, Frequency And Vibration"*
>
> — NIKOLA TESLA

This may be the most important part of the book for you to truly grasp because your recovery is not just about fixing what's "broken", it's about connecting into the boundless energy field that surrounds you and exists within you. The fact is that most people look at the world in a linear way. **They think that the A + B = C.** That if I do X then I will get Y. That's simply not how things work. A + B can equal Y or A + B can also equal 5. **The universe works in mysterious and unpredictable ways**, in ways that we will never be able to understand reality completely. Science and traditional physics do help. And they do explain a lot about reality, but they can't ever explain everything. That is impossible. A lot of this comes from the way we were raised to perceive the world. I mean, look at the stars. The light that you see has taken millions of light years to get here. When we look above, we can also see that most of the sky is made up of darkness. A similar discovery happened when scientists used **transmission elec-tron microscopes** to see what is going inside of **subatomic particles. Bear with me, if an ex-college dropout** can learn this, then so can you. Atoms appear to be 99.99999999999 percent empty space. But that space isn't really empty. It's actually filled with **energy and infor-mation.** This is exactly what Einstein called "Spooky Action at a Distance."

I need to tell you about the experiment conducted by Nicolas Gisin, a physicist who explored the realm of quantum entanglement. In his groundbreaking research, Gisin and his team separated two entangled atoms. What's mind-blowing is that these atoms communicated with each other faster than the speed of light, a phenomenon that defies our everyday understanding of how things "should work". When one atom was affected, the other atom responded instantly, regardless of the distance between them. This experiment demonstrates that everything in the universe is interconnected in ways we don't fully understand. The energy exchanged between those atoms reveals a deeper truth about reality that we are all part of a vast, interconnected energy field.

After a brain injury, it's common to feel like your energy has been drained and your spirit dimmed. But the truth is, your energy has not left you, it's simply been disrupted. You have the power to shift your state, elevate your vibration, and tap into a level of healing that goes beyond just physical recovery. It's about accessing a higher consciousness where true transformation happens. Energy is the foundation of everything, the invisible force that shapes your reality fuels your healing and rewires your brain.

I want to tell a story to you all, and maybe you can relate. It feels like yesterday, as I was sitting on the floor of my room. I was feeling quite awful at the time. I decided that I would not get up from the meditation until I felt much better. In the months prior to this, there was something that really bugged me. I often asked myself if I was developing Parkinson's disease, like the great Muhammad Ali. **It tortured me to my core.** After 30-45 minutes into the meditation, my head started shaking quite violently and rapidly. It was really scary! Like violent, super random convulsions. The intensity only continued to get more and more. However, I decided to stop fighting the shaking. Let go and trust that this was "supposed" to be happening. I continued to shake violently, maybe even more forceful than before for about 2-3 minutes. When I did that, I experienced a huge energy release that to this day is difficult to describe. The best way I can say it, I felt a huge trauma release and a deep connection to the Universe. It was as if space and time collapsed upon itself.

I have had multiple experiences like this during my meditation. **Needless to say, I have never doubted the power of energy since then. Because that is all that there is!**

For you, this means that your recovery isn't just a linear process. By tapping into this energy, connecting with your surroundings, and engaging with your inner self, you can ignite a transformation that goes beyond just healing. You can *generate* a new reality filled with possibility. The energy you generate within yourself can transcend barriers, much like the atoms in Gisin's experiment. This powerful connection can lead you to new heights in your journey toward recovery and wholeness. Embrace it and watch your life transform.

Action Step: Three Easy Steps to Interrupt Your Pattern!!!

When you get stuck in an unproductive way of thinking, feeling, acting, or overall bad energetic state, you really need to break the pattern. At the end of the day, **every action has an equal and opposite reaction in the universe.** Call this the law of karma or whatever you want to call it, "it" is undeniably true!

1. Catch yourself! Whenever you have a negative thought, emotion, or behavior, catch yourself and become aware of it. For extra effect, you can scream out or yell out in your mind, "STOP".
2. Interrupt the pattern. Depending on how strong, hardwired, or automatic the pattern is, you will need to interrupt it with an equally powerful force. Some of the best ways to interrupt the pattern are to take a deep breath when you say something negative. Other ways are to take a cold shower, engage in vigorous exercise, change your environment, or a continuous deep cyclical hyperventilation breathing.
3. Repeat! Things often do not change after one time of interrupting the pattern. Continue to do this until it breaks the pattern for good!

Claim Your VIP Spot Today! Get early access to discounts, offers, and 15 free Mind Gym exercises. Just scan the QR code or go to www.dr-bro.com/vipbrainrescue.

CHAPTER SIX: THE THIRD PILLAR: B IS FOR B.R.A.I.N

This section is all about the 5 principles of Neuroplasticity to use for predictable results in your memory recovery journey. When you harness the five core principles of neuroplasticity—Breathing, Repetition, Association, Intensity, and Novelty—you unlock your brain's full potential to recover your memory and thrive. These 5 core principles are not only a matter of neuroscience, but ultimately a matter of the laws of physics.

THE FIRST STEP IS B FOR BREATHING:

> *"Breath is the bridge which connects life to consciousness, which unites your body to your thoughts."*
>
> — THÍCH NHẤT HẠNH

Breathing matters! Breathing is the essence of all life. Your brain, which makes up only 2% of your body mass, consumes 20% of your body's energy. To activate your brain properly, you need to master the skill of intentional breathing. The way you breathe matters a lot.

Here is the thing. When you breathe in you are activating your sympathetic nervous system. When you breathe out you are relaxing your parasympathetic system. If you are a shallow breather, you prevent the parasympathetic system from engaging properly. As a result, stress hormones flood your system, clouding your thinking and activating your primal survival response. Fast, shallow, and mouth/breathing = anxiety. Deep breathing causes your abdomen to rise and fall and consequently, lowers your heart rate. When you breathe deeply, your body naturally shifts into a state of calm. Meaning, you can literally shift your state with breath.

The inhalation portion of the breath is energizing—the exhalations are relaxing. In the same way that your heart rate/breathing rate changes according to your state. [24]

Where the breath goes, energy and blood flow go. Better blood flow means better brain health. Think about if a lion walked in the door behind you, you wouldn't be taking a long exhale. You would be ready to run your ass off. Deep breathing engages the diaphragm, which is closely linked to the vagus nerve. Breathing is directly correlated to memory recall. Meaning that your breathing patterns influence how well you remember things.

In the world with my patients, we explore and quantify different skills like **Breath Holds** and **CO_2 tolerance training** to build stress resilience, improve oxygenation, and create an ideal environment for memory restoration. By adjusting the pace and intensity of your breathing, you can change your brain's state, reduce stress, and improve cognitive function fast!

Now, let's dive into the incredible science behind **Breath Holds.**

But before we dive into that, have you watched the movie "The Waterboy" with Adam Sandler playing the role of Bobby Boucher? I don't know if you love it, but I do, and you need to check it out. There is a hilarious scene with a professor who looks like Colonel Sanders who asks his class, "**Can anyone tell me why alligators are so** aggressive all the time?" Boucher raises his hand and says, "**Momma says it because alligators got all their teeth but no way to brush them!**" The class laughs and another student raises his hand and says, "Alligators are so aggressive because of the size of their medulla oblongata." Boucher yells out in disbelief and storms out of the class in defense of his momma. Eventually, the Professor says, "Something must be wrong with his medulla oblongata!" Sandler loses his mind in anger and tackles the professor.

Ironically, **the medulla oblongata is a very important area of self-regulation**. And you can activate its neuroplasticity through breath holds. It plays a role in regulating autonomic functions such as heart rate, breathing, and reflexes. Breath control techniques, including breath holds, can indeed help improve aspects of autonomic regulation by influencing the nervous system, and the medulla oblongata itself is just one part of this complex process.

It is a skill that most people never tap into. That's exactly what happens when you practice **breath holds**. You're not just holding your breath—you're waking up your brain's **chemoreceptors** in the medulla oblongata, the control center in your brainstem that monitors CO_2 levels. [25]

As CO_2 builds up, these sensors trigger powerful signals, forcing your brain to adapt and grow stronger. This isn't just about breathing—it's about building resilience. By training your body to handle stress and increasing your CO_2 tolerance, you're training your brain to stay calm under pressure and to perform at its absolute best. Holding your breath is one of the most effective and efficient things you can do to build your stress tolerance. Think about it. There is nothing more stressful than the lack of oxygen.

Here's the kicker: this process fuels neuroplasticity, your brain's ability to rewire itself. You're creating the perfect conditions for your brain and memory to heal, grow, and perform at levels you didn't think were possible. This is life-changing stuff, you're literally reprogramming your brain's ability to recover and thrive. This isn't just about holding your breath—it's your brain's secret weapon to better health. Just as you need to practice the mechanics of shooting a great jump shot, you will understand how changing the pace and intensity of your breathing can rapidly change the state of your brain health. Holding your breath allows you to tap into the zero-point field, where the past, present and future all simultaneously exist.

ACTION STEP:

Try This 3-Step Breath Hold Secret:

Step 1: Cyclical Hyperventilation Breathing

Start by sitting comfortably. Take 30 very deep, steady breaths to flood your body with adrenaline and oxygen. Breathe by expanding your belly. Steady powerful inhales through your mouth. This primes your lungs and makes it easier to hold your breath for longer.

Step 2: The Breath Hold

On your last deep inhale, take a full breath and hold. Stay calm as your CO_2 levels rise. This is where your brain starts to adapt and grow stronger. Hold for as long as you can without straining, then exhale slowly.

Step 3: Build Your Strength

Rest for a minute, then repeat for 3-5 rounds. With each round, push yourself to hold your breath just a little longer. This not only builds CO_2 tolerance but trains your brain to handle stress, boosting your recovery.

Step 4: Track Your Results and Repeat.

It's important to time how long you can hold your breath, so that you can see the improvements over time.

THE SECOND STEP IS R FOR REPETITION:

> "Repetition Is The Mother Of Learning, The Father Of Action, Which Makes It The Architect Of Accomplishment."
>
> — ZIG ZIGLAR

Repetition matters! It's not just a nice-to-know fact; it's a universal truth and the driving force behind all change. **Repetition is the mother of all learning. What we repeat, we become better at ... period!** This timeless adage holds especially true in the context of **memory** recovery after a concussion or brain injury. Why? When the brain is damaged, the old communication pathways, those routes your brain relies on to function, get disrupted. Neuroplasticity is triggered by consistent, deliberate action. When you're on the battlefield of brain injury recovery, **repetition is your best friend.**

Let me explain.

My friend Quintero, who's deep into his studies to become a clinical neuroscientist, put it perfectly: **"When you have a brain injury, essentially you have a disruption in the pathways your brain uses to solve common problems to accomplish a goal."**

Think about that. Whether it's the goal of **thinking, speaking, moving,** or anything else—those smooth, automatic brain functions you once had are now suddenly interrupted. **It's like hitting a construction roadblock or detour!** Your brain has to find a new longer pathway to solve the same problem or achieve the same goal. Whatever that goal is, like tying your shoes, talking, walking, whatever that is! It takes lots of time and energy for the brain to rewire.

Look at the diagrams below to see exactly what I mean.

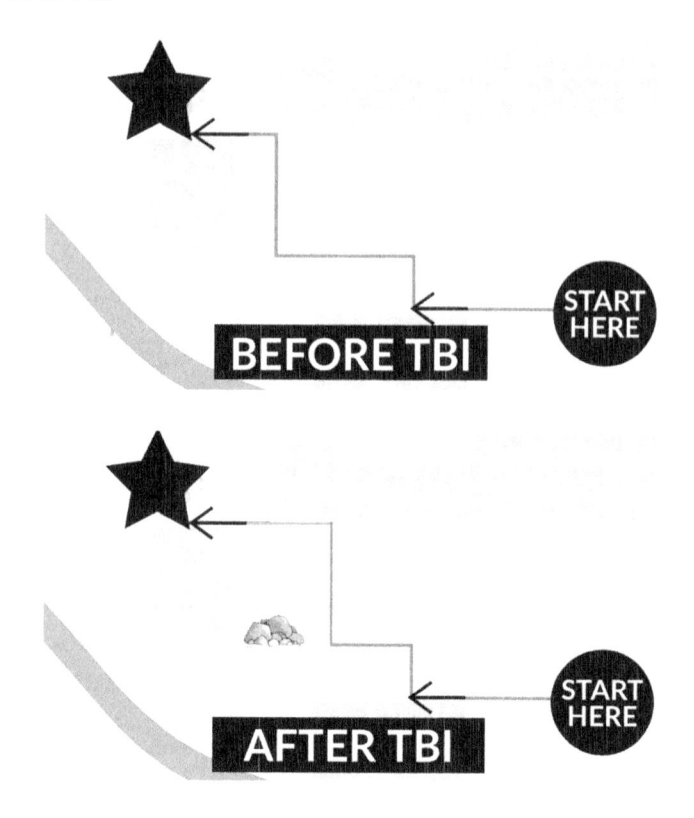

Your brain's like a highway. Before the injury, you're flying down the fast lane, no problem. But after the injury? Boom. It's like a wreck hits—roads are blocked, and detours are everywhere. What used to be easy is now a grind. But here's the thing: your brain can't sit around waiting for the roads to clear. It has to build new ones. It has to form new pathways to solve the same problems it did before.

And how do you do that? **Repetition.** Every day, you take that new route, and yeah, at first, it sucks, it's slow and frustrating. But if you keep at it, it will become easier. Eventually, that new path becomes your best path. It will become automatic. That's how you rebuild. That's how you win.

Your brain is really smart. The more you repeat a behavior your brain will say "**Hey! You keep doing this thing?** I am going to create an automatic pattern, so that you don't have to waste energy thinking about how to do this thing. I'll just have you do this thing!"

Know that it's not just about repetition and pattern of habit. It's also about patterns and habits of thought. Those habitual thinking patterns we have can either empower or disempower us.

When you think or behave in some way, you are firing and wiring specific brain cells growing and connecting together. And by doing so your brain is saving more energy as it automates the process. **Repetition is a simple concept but not easy to apply.** Habits aren't formed by doing something just once. They're built through consistent repetition. Think about how you learned to walk, speak, brush your teeth or memorize your times tables — these skills became second nature because you practiced them repeatedly. The same principle applies to the way we think. Repetition shapes habits, and it's one of the key reasons many people struggle to improve their memory.

Be patient and trust in the process. Once again, science shows that building a new neural network takes 60 to 254 days to become an automatic habit. Much like it takes a long time to build a new road.

Remember, my friend, practice doesn't make perfect. Practice makes progress, and then eventually, practice makes permanent. Meaning that it becomes so automatic the pathways in your brain will lead you in the right direction without needing you to focus or concentrate.

THE THIRD STEP IS A FOR ASSOCIATION:

> "Surround Yourself With People Who Are Going To Lift You Higher."
>
> — OPRAH

Association Matters! Association is how our brain connects and makes sense of the world around us. Changing your associations are how you change your perception of your recovery because perception is reality. Your brain builds connections between ideas, memories, and emotions through associations, which helps you make sense of the world. Think of it this way: if repetition is the hammer that forges new pathways, then association is the glue that holds everything together. When you link new information to something you already know or care about, you create stronger, longer-lasting memories. It's not just about recalling facts—it's about connecting them to your life. For example, when you think of the phrase "**New York City,**" what comes to mind? For me, it brings up **images** of the **Empire State Building, Statue of Liberty, Pizza, and Hotdogs.** Now, consider the word "**hot dog.**" What do you associate with it? Perhaps you think of ketchup, relish, or a bustling hot dog stand. **This is how our brains make meaning of the world around us, often without us even realizing it.** In the context of **memory** recovery, the law of association becomes even more critical. After a concussion or brain injury, the pathways your brain usually relies on to retrieve memories may be weakened, stretched, or damaged.

Be Careful of Who You Surround Yourself With

You may have heard the saying, "**You are the average of the five people you spend the most time with.**" This means that your beliefs, thoughts, actions, habits, and hobbies can be influenced by those around you. Therefore, it's essential to be mindful of your associations. I can tell you that the people you hang out with will either uplift or bring you down.

I can't stress this enough! In high school and my early twenties, **I fell in with the wrong crowd.** It started innocently enough hanging out, listening to rap music, going to parties. At first, it felt exciting, even harmless. I was still on track, graduating high school and doing well in college. But as time went on, I noticed a subtle shift. The influence of the people I surrounded myself with began to creep into my life. **Without realizing it**, I started adopting their mindset—their beliefs, attitudes, and even their values. What I thought was harmless fun began to lead me down a path of chaos. It's remarkable how powerful external influences can be. The more time I spent in that circle, the more I began to think and act like them. **The music we blasted wasn't just background noise; it was shaping my world view.** The people I thought were just friends were, in fact, reshaping my priorities. Looking back, I see it clearly: who you spend your time with doesn't just influence you, it defines you. Consider how you perceive important topics **like money, health, and self-image.** If you're trying to remember a new concept, tie it to something meaningful to you—such as a personal story, a specific place, or a particular feeling. This strategy is how you build memories that truly stick. Through understanding the power of association, you can actively shape your **memory** recovery and personal growth. Remember that your brain is adaptable; it can learn and form new connections. **Embrace this journey** and be intentional about the associations you create.

Pavlov's Dog: Woof Woof. Use the Law of Association

Pavlov's dog teaches us a powerful lesson about how our brains learn and how law of association works.

Here's a quick overview:

Stage 1: The Dog and the Food

In the first stage, Ivan Pavlov presented food to his dog, which caused it to drool—a natural, automatic reaction known as an "unconditioned response."

Stage 2: Introducing the Bell

Next, Pavlov rang a bell before giving the dog food. At first, the dog didn't care about the bell. However, after repeated pairings of the bell and food, the dog began to associate the two together.

Stage 3: The Dog Learns

Eventually, the dog drooled at the sound of the bell alone, demonstrating a "conditioned response." It learned to expect food from the bell, much like how you might feel excitement when your phone buzzes.

Stage 4: The Bell Alone

When Pavlov rang the bell without food, the dog still drooled, showing a strong connection between the bell and food. However, if this continued without food, the response eventually faded, this is called "extinction."

Why This Matters to You

Our brains, like Pavlov's dog, learn through patterns and associations. For example, after dealing with headaches after a concussion, you might feel stressed if you hear the word "recovery." But by practicing positive techniques and affirmation, you can retrain your brain to associate recovery with feeling better.

Check out the diagram below for more reference. (Photo credit to tyonote)

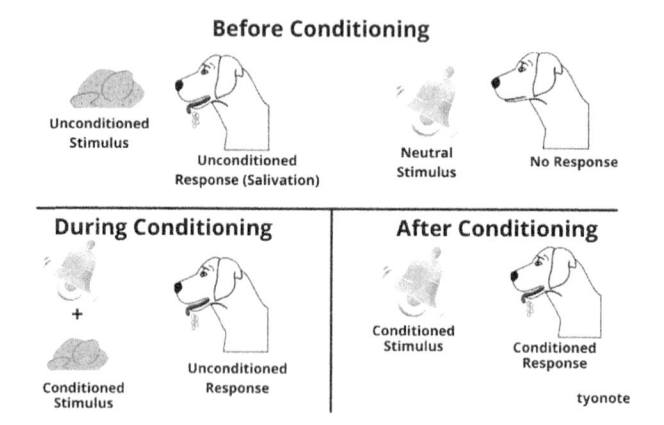

Before Conditioning

Unconditioned Stimulus — Unconditioned Response (Salivation)

Neutral Stimulus — No Response

During Conditioning

Conditioned Stimulus + Unconditioned Response

After Conditioning

Conditioned Stimulus — Conditioned Response

tyonote

Taking Action: 5 Steps to Activate the Power of Association in Your Recovery.

1. **Create a Mind Map:** Visualize connections by drawing a mind map. Write down a central idea (like "recovery") and branch out with associated memories, feelings, and experiences. This can help reinforce the connections in your mind.
2. **Link New Information to Personal Stories:** Whenever you learn something new, ask yourself how it relates to your own life. This could be a memory, an experience, or even a goal. For instance, if you learn about healthy eating, think back to a time when you felt great after a nutritious meal.
3. **Use Visual Aids:** Incorporate images, symbols, or even objects that represent the ideas you want to remember. For example, place a picture of a balanced meal on your fridge as a reminder of your commitment to health.
4. **Practice Positive Affirmations:** Reinforce your new associations with daily affirmations. If you're working on recovery, repeat phrases like "I am making progress every day" or "I am resilient." These affirmations can help shift your mindset and strengthen your mental connections.
5. **Surround Yourself with Supportive People:** Seek out friends, family, or support groups that foster positive associations. Engaging with others who inspire you can enhance your belief in your ability to recover and thrive.

THE FOURTH STEP IS I FOR INTENSITY:

> *"Without Intensity, Passion Fades. It's The Driving Force That Fuels Achievement."*
>
> — BRUCE LEE

Intensity Matters! Listen up. The fact that you are reading this book, is an indication that you are a knowledge seeker. You've already taken the first step by admitting you need to change. That alone speaks volumes about your courage and willingness to grow. Change starts with a spark. Desire alone won't get you there. True transformation comes from consistent effort, focus, and yes, intensity. **Intensity isn't about hoping for results or wishing your way out of your prob-lems.** It's about quitting the doubt, eliminating excuses, and creating the person you want to become. If you want to evolve, here's what's important showing up with your whole heart. Remember, discom-fort and resistance isn't always something to fear. In fact, they can be signs that you are stretching and growing. When things get tough, and they will, that can be a sign to lean in. Push gently past your limits to find strength you didn't know you had. The journey isn't about pushing yourself past your limits or "toughing it out." It's about building trust within yourself and proving that you can rise to the challenge. **So, take a deep breath.** When you feel the challenge, when your mind tells you to stop, that's the moment to dig a little deeper. That's when you prove to yourself that you're stronger than you thought, a true Warrior!

The Intensity Science

Now, let's peel back the neuroscience behind **intensity. Your brain responds to high-energy, emotionally charged experiences.** When you learn something with intensity, whether it's pushing yourself in a tough workout or diving into an exciting new challenge, it leaves a deeper mark. The emotional energy activates your amygdala, strengthening the memory. So, if you're trying to make something unforgettable, don't just go through the motions; pour your energy into it. Treat each practice like you're going for a win, not just putting in time. This turns ordinary learning into extraordinary progress. **When you crank up the intensity, your brain is firing on all cylinders!** The prefrontal cortex acts as your game-day coach, keeping your decisions sharp and focused, while the anterior cingulate cortex drives your determination to push through tough moments. The parietal cortex heightens your awareness, filtering out distractions, with the thalamus acting as your brain's bouncer, letting only the most important signals through. The basal ganglia pumps out dopamine, motivating you to keep grinding, and the amygdala channels your emotions into fuel, turning fear into focus. Your hippocampus strengthens your memory, locking in lessons learned from intense experiences, while the insula connects feelings to attention, helping you tune into your body's signals. Finally, the cerebellum fine-tunes your movements and thoughts, ensuring precision in everything you do. **So when you bring the heat, you're not just working hard; you're transforming your brain into the dream team ready to conquer any challenge!**

THE FIFTH STEP IS N FOR NOVELTY:

> *"Novelty Is The Mother Of Attraction. It Stimulates Us, Intrigues us, and draws us in."*
>
> — DAVID LIEBERMAN

Novelty matters! Novelty means anything new to us. That can be as small as reading a new idea, or as big as taking a life-changing trip to Africa! Novelty keeps our brains excited, sharp, and on our toes. It

doesn't matter how big or small it is; what matters is that it shakes you out of your routine and gets those neurons firing. When you expose yourself to new experiences, your brain releases dopamine, the feel-good neurotransmitter that also plays a massive role in learning and memory. Don't be booooring! You want to remember something better? Do new things! When your brain associates a new experience with that rush of dopamine, it's like putting a neon sign in your memory: "Remember this!" This is especially important if you're dealing with memory issues after a concussion or brain injury. You've got to create new pathways, and novelty is your best tool for the job. So, what does that look like in practice? It means getting out of your comfort zone.

Challenge Yourself Daily!

Read that book you've been eyeing, try a new workout routine, or immerse yourself in a completely different culture. Even the little things matter. Take a different route to work, learn a new recipe, or explore a hobby you've never considered. The goal is to keep your brain engaged and hungry for more.

It's a powerful strategy for healing and growth. The more you feed your brain with new experiences, the more adaptable and resilient you become. You're not just surviving; you're actively thriving, transforming your challenges into strengths.

So, get out there! Seek out novelty, embrace the new, and unleash the full potential of your brain. This is your journey, and you're the one in control. Make it count!

Action Step: Explore a New Commute

It's time to break the monotony. Take a different route to work today —train, car, or bus, it doesn't matter. Bonus points if you don't use GPS and use a good old-fashioned map. This isn't just about getting from point A to B; you're firing up your parietal lobe, sharpening your mind, and memory. Plus, you will get to see new things you haven't seen before.

Now you've got the blueprint to sharpen your memory, and it's as simple as B.R.A.I.N. **Breathing, Repetition, Association, Intensity, and Novelty.** Now it's time to take action—start small, stay consistent, and let your brain's true potential explode. You've got this.

MAKE A DIFFERENCE

"The Best Way To Find Yourself Is To Lose Yourself In The Service Of Others."

— MAHATMA GANDHI

Helping others is one of the most powerful ways to find fulfillment. When we give freely, without expecting anything in return, we not only help others but also enrich our own lives. Together, we can make a difference. If you're someone who has experienced the journey of healing after a brain injury, you know how damn challenging it can be. But you also know the power of taking small, meaningful steps toward recovery. I wrote *Brain Rescue* to make brain recovery easy and achievable for everyone, especially those who might feel overwhelmed or unsure where to begin.

But to truly reach more people, I need your help.

When someone is looking for guidance, they often turn to reviews to see if a book is right for them. That's where you come in! By leaving a review, you can make a huge difference in someone's life.

It only takes a minute, but your words could change someone's path to recovery. Your review might just help:

- One more person regain hope after a brain injury.
- One more person start their journey to healing with guidance and confidence.
- One more person discover that a holistic brain recovery is possible.

To leave a review, simply scan the QR code below and share your thoughts:

Thank you so much for your support. Your generosity means the world to me and to everyone who will benefit from your words.

With gratitude,

Dr. Bro

CHAPTER SEVEN: THE FOURTH PILLAR: O IS FOR O.P.T.I.M.I.Z.E

We're now entering a critical and exciting stage in your recovery that goes beyond simply restoring your brain to its former state. This is about **OPTIMIZING** your cognitive function to levels you may have never dreamed possible.

OPTIMISM: Your Mind's Superpower for Healing and Growth

THE FIRST STEP IS O FOR OPTIMISM:

> *"Between Stimulus And Response, There Is A Space. In That Space Is Our Power To Choose Our Response. In Our Response Lies Our Growth And Our Freedom."*
>
> — VIKTOR FRANKL

Optimism a major key to optimization. When it comes to optimizing your brain, one factor stands out above all others: Optimism. It's not just about feeling good; it's about unleashing a biological force within you that can drive healing, growth, and transformation. **Did you know that just one optimistic thought can produce more than**

30,000 neurochemicals at a moment's notice? That's right. Your brain is wired to respond powerfully to optimism. It is, without a doubt, the most potent pharmacy you have at your disposal, capable of releasing natural chemicals that boost your mood, sharpen your focus, and accelerate your recovery. Optimism isn't just wishful thinking. It's your superpower! [26] Cultivating a positive mindset is step one if you ever want to maximize your brain potential. Without it is like building a skyscraper with no foundation. Even if you do all the "right things", like eating healthy, exercising, and meditating. But, if you are doing those out of fear, instead of inspiration, you might as well stop.

Start By Smiling

As **Dr. Andrew Huberman** would explain, the science behind it is called "facial feedback," meaning when you move those facial muscles, you're not just showing emotion—you're creating it. The signals travel from your face to the reward centers of the brain, flipping the switch from stress to calmness, from anxiety to optimism. It's not just a superficial act; you're hacking your brain to turn on the systems responsible for feeling good, staying focused, and bouncing back faster.

Celebrate The Small Things

I want you to begin celebrating all of the "small wins" in your life. Now it may seem counterintuitive at first, but really it is the the key to creating more discipline in your life. Let me tell you that discipline is powerful, but it does no good if you aren't enjoying the process. If you only rely on discipline and consistency, without a sense of optimism, you will burn out! It's only a matter of time. The truth is that small wins stack up to become big wins and breakthroughs in your life. Once again, think of it as if you are climbing a big icy, snowy mountain in the Himalayas. Climbing to the top is your goal of getting a **sharp memory** and an optimized brain. When you climb a mountain, you really have to take it one step at a time. If you get too preoccupied with looking too far up or down the mountain, that can be distracting. Sometimes, there will be storms coming, and sometimes, you will slip down the ice, causing a setback.

This is normal in the recovery process. There will be good days and bad days. But, if you take it one step at a time and begin to celebrate the small wins, you will look back on all the progress you've made! I'm not a fan of the term brain hacks, but if there were ever such a thing as a hack it would be getting into the frequency of celebration.

I mean something as basic as brushing your teeth, taking a walk or finishing a workout.

Really get into it! Don't hold back! Dance! Give high fives, yell out YES! Even if there is no one around to celebrate. With time practicing this will become an automatic part of your routine and will pay off huge with time. If you aren't able to appreciate the small stuff, you will **NEVER EVER** be able to appreciate the big moments of life.

THE SECOND STEP IS P FOR PROCESSING:

> *The Human Brain Is A Complex And Delicate System, Capable Of Processing An Unimaginable Amount Of Information In A Split Second."*
>
> — DAVID EAGLEMAN

Processing is another important step to unlocking the door to your brain's potential. Doing so will dramatically transform your **memory**, focus, and overall mental performance.

What is Brain Processing and Why Does It Matter?

Think of processing as the way your brain makes sense of everything coming at it. It is how it organizes, stores, and retrieves information.

Cars buzzing by, people talking, and mind-numbing construction noises. All kinds of sights, tastes, sounds, smells, and vibrations.

All this input is like a flood of data that your brain must quickly sort out and make sense of.

It has to rapidly answer questions, "Have I seen this before? Am I safe?

After it has done all that, it now has to make a decision based on all input it has received.

Now you may be beginning to understand how important the ability to process really is.

It's estimated that the human brain takes in an astonishing 11 million bits of information per second from all of your senses. [27] [28] **Luckily, our brain only keeps us consciously or intently aware of a very small percentage of that.** The ability to process this information quickly and accurately is crucial for performing everyday tasks, remembering details, and staying mentally sharp.

When processing slows down after a brain injury or concussion, **it can feel like your mind is in a fog**, and even simple tasks may seem difficult. This phenomenon, commonly known as "brain fog," occurs because the brain's ability to quickly and efficiently handle information has been impaired. After a head injury, the brain experiences a **disruption** in its normal functioning, leading to difficulties with tasks that used to be easy, such as reading, holding a conversation, or even making a simple grocery list. The slowed processing speed can make it challenging to follow along with **fast paced world.**

But what if I could tell you that with practice, we can not only improve things but get them to a higher level than you ever have experienced before?

How to Improve Processing Speed? Here Are 3 Dynamic Ways

1. **Meditation.** You may have heard about the benefits of meditation for relaxation, but did you know that it can significantly enhance your brain's processing capabilities too? Studies have shown that regular meditation practice increases gray matter density in brain regions associated with **memory,** attention, and processing speed.[29] It essentially trains your mind to operate more efficiently by reducing distractions and enhancing your ability to focus. Even just 10-15 minutes a day can lead to noticeable improvements in how quickly you can take in and respond to information. **Meditation is much more than just a stress-relief tool; it's a scientifically proven method to build a stronger, more resilient brain.** Incorporating techniques like mindfulness or focused breathing can not only help you calm your nervous system but also stimulate new neural pathways that enhance the speed at which your brain processes information.

2. **Eye saccades** are quick movements your eyes make when you shift focus from one point to another. Think of them like the way your eyes jump around when you read or look at different things around you. These movements are super important for helping your brain process what you see. When you practice exercises that improve your eye movements, you can train your brain to take in information faster and more efficiently. **By exercising eye movements, you're helping your brain become faster at processing visual information.**[30]

3. **Speed reading techniques** are designed to help you absorb written information more rapidly, without sacrificing comprehension. By learning to take in information in larger chunks and **eliminating the habit of subvocalization**

(saying words silently as you read), you can train your brain to process written content more quickly. This directly helps improve processing speed, as it forces your brain to keep up with the faster reading pace, which strengthens pathways involved in comprehension and memory. Apply these skills to your daily life and notice the changes.

THE THIRD STEP IS T FOR TIMING:

> *"It's Not The Strongest Or The Smartest Who Survive, But Those Who Can Respond Most Quickly."*
>
> — CHARLES DARWIN

I'm not a big fan of Darwin and his teachings but I do love that quote. To really get your brain on track, we will discuss the power of timing—more specifically, reaction timing. Think of your brain like a phone. Reaction timing is how quickly it responds when you tap the screen—instant and smooth. Processing speed is the power behind the scenes, making sure everything loads fast without lag. However, reaction timing isn't about speed; it's about precision and how quickly you can retrieve and apply what you know in real-time. It isn't just something you inherit—it's a weapon you can forge. Think of reaction timing as the brain's "readiness system." When fine-tuned, your brain becomes quicker at recalling information and making decisions on the fly. This section is about mastering the power of reaction timing to boost memory and brain function to its fullest potential.

Why Reaction Timing Matters For Memory

The faster your brain can react, the more efficient the **memory** pathways become, making responses automatic. This isn't a coincidence; memory and reaction timing are highly linked. When your reaction timing is sharp, your brain is primed to process information quickly and respond efficiently. Every time you react to something—a movement, a question, a mental challenge—your brain relies on complex memory circuits and precise timing to fire the right response. **Studies show that faster reaction time means better cognitive flexibility** (the ability to switch between thoughts or tasks smoothly), which is a key component of strong **memory.** By training your brain's reaction timing, you create stronger and faster neural connections, making it easier to retrieve information when you need it. [31] It's about building a brain that works fluidly, able to remember, analyze, and act all in a split second. Let's dive into how you can optimize this skill to improve your brain's health, resilience, and memory.

How Working Memory and Reaction Timing Work Together

Working memory is like a mental notepad, holding information we need to use right away—whether it's directions or facts for a test. Reaction timing is how quickly we respond to things happening around us. When you improve your reaction timing, your brain gets faster at pulling information from working memory. Studies show that reaction-time training also strengthens working memory. For example, research published in Frontiers in Human Neuroscience found that people who trained their reaction timing could remember things more easily. [32] Simply put, the faster your reaction timing, the quicker and better your brain can remember and use information.

Training Reaction Timing

- **Visual Reaction Timing:** Over 70% of the brain's real estate is dedicated to vision. Enhancing your visual reaction time can significantly improve your overall cognitive function and memory. Improving visual reaction timing strengthens pathways in the occipital lobe for visual processing, enhancing spatial awareness in the parietal lobe, and coordinating reactions to visual stimuli through the superior colliculus. This includes simple drills, like catching a ball or peripheral training. [33]

2. **Auditory (Sound) Reaction Timing**: Improving auditory reaction timing improves processing speed as well. The enhancement strengthens several brain regions. It improves sound processing in the auditory cortex, boosts language comprehension in Wernicke's area, and supports quick responses to sounds through the brainstem. Engaging in activities such as rhythm exercises or auditory drills can effectively develop this skill. [34]

3. **Physical (Kinesthetic) Reaction Timing**: Enhancing kinesthetic reaction timing is crucial for improving your body's response to physical movements. This skill is linked to the motor cortex, which controls voluntary movements, as well as the cerebellum, responsible for balance and coordination. Training in physical activities—such as agility drills, sports, or dance—can significantly improve your kinesthetic reaction timing. By focusing on these activities, you can boost your body's ability to react quickly and efficiently, enhancing overall coordination and athletic performance.

Take Action! Color, Call, Catch

What You Need:

- A set of colored balls (like red, blue, green, etc.) or colored paper balls (you can make these easily).
- A partner (or you can do it alone with colored paper).

Instructions:

1. **Set Up:**
   - If you have a partner, stand about 10 feet apart. If you're alone, just spread the colored balls out on the ground in front of you.
2. **The Game:**
   - **Auditory:** One player (the caller) will call out a color (like "Red!").
   - **Visual:** Look for the ball of that color as quickly as you can.
   - **Physical:** When you see the ball of the called color, run and catch it or pick it up.
3. **How to Play:**
   - The caller can mix it up by calling out different colors quickly or even making silly sounds to keep you on your toes.
   - If you're playing alone, just call out the color yourself and see how fast you can react!
4. **Repeat:**
   - Keep playing for about 5–10 minutes, changing colors frequently to keep it exciting.

THE FOURTH STEP IS I FOR INHIBITION:

> *"Your New Life is Going to Cost Your Old One!"*
>
> — WES WATSON

Inhibition, from a neurological standpoint, is the ability to inhibit, suppress, or restrain brain activity. This step will be longer than many others because it is extremely overlooked and important to your successful recovery! When it comes to self-improvement, most people know that action is important. And it is! But what they fail to recognize is that what we choose to NO longer do is equally important. Understand that Hebb's law states that **neurons that fire together, wire together.** But also, **neurons that no longer fire together no longer wire together....**

Brain cells and connections grow depending on what you do! And they also atrophy or shrink depending on what you no longer choose to do!!!

It's really that simple!

It's hard to understand why the ability to inhibit (stop) behavior is so overlooked. It is equally important to the recovery process as activation.

Did you know there are over 100 chemicals hard at work at any given time in your brain?

These chemical messengers influence and transmit everything from your emotions to movement.

Types of Neurotransmitters: Activation vs Inhibition

Neurochemicals can generally be categorized into two types of categories.

Excitatory (Activating) Neurochemicals and Inhibitory (Calming) Neurochemicals.

There can be further broken into three subcategories of neurochemicals.

Don't let this confuse you if you are at the beginning level.

Neurotransmitters, Neuromodulators, and Neuropeptides aka Neurohormones

Neurotransmitters are like messengers that send signals between brain cells, helping control things like mood and movement.

Neuromodulators help adjust how neurotransmitters work, like turning up or down the volume on a radio to change how strong the signals are.

Neuropeptides/Neurohormones are special messengers that travel through your body and control bigger things, like hunger or stress. For instance, endorphins help you feel good after exercise.

Think of each neurochemical like a worker in a busy factor, with each that has its own important job.

List of Excitatory (Activating) Chemicals

These are essential for increasing mental alertness, motivation, energy, and cognitive function.

- **Glutamate** – The primary excitatory neurotransmitter, crucial for learning, memory, and overall brain function.
- **Dopamine** – Central to the brain's reward system; influences motivation, pleasure, and focus.
- **Norepinephrine** (Noradrenaline) – Enhances attention, alertness, and response to stress.
- **Serotonin** – Primarily a mood stabilizer but can also promote wakefulness and focus.
- **Acetylcholine** – Vital for learning, memory, and muscle activation; plays an excitatory role in many parts of the brain.
- **Histamine** – Involved in wakefulness and alertness, as well as immune responses.
- **Phenylethylamine (PEA)** – Increases energy and focus; associated with feelings of excitement and euphoria.

List of Inhibitory (Calming) Neurotransmitters

- **GABA** (Gamma-Aminobutyric Acid) – The primary inhibitory neurotransmitter, reducing neural activity to promote calm.

- **Glycine** – Calms neural activity, especially in the spinal cord, supporting stability and relaxation.
- **Adenosine** – Builds up during wakefulness, promoting sleep and relaxation.
- **Melatonin** – Regulates circadian rhythms, supporting relaxation and sleep.
- **Endocannabinoids** (like Anandamide) – Calms stress and reduces pain, supporting emotional balance.

The War Within

One of the biggest issues most people experience after a head injury is **impulsiveness**. It was a huge problem for me as well. **I just couldn't say no to anyone or anything!**. Whether that was drugs, alcohol, or food. I grew to 195 pounds (88 kilos). I felt miserable at that weight. Did my seizure medications play a role? Absolutely, but it was mostly down to how my brain was functioning. Impulsiveness nearly destroyed my life on many different occasions. From abusing and selling hard drugs, getting in a fight with a bouncer, getting arrested for public drunkenness in the Dominican Republic, falling asleep on the sidewalk, and getting robbed at gunpoint. I could go on and on. Not to glorify, but I want you to learn from me and not go down the pathway I did.

For me, impulsiveness wasn't just an inconvenience; it was war! I can't tell you how many times I felt powerless, unable to fight against those sudden urges. And I know a lot of you reading this have been there. It's like you're standing outside your body, watching yourself make decisions you *know* aren't right, but you feel completely incapable of stopping them.

Impulsiveness nearly destroyed my life on many different occasions. A smart person learns from their own mistakes, but a wise one learns from the mistakes of others. As George W. Bush once said, "Fool me once, shame on you, fool me twice, you not gonna fool me again!"

Why Brain Injuries Disrupt Impulse Control

To understand how **inhibition** breaks down after a brain injury, we need to talk about the frontal lobe. As mentioned before, most brain injuries take place at the front of the head. The front part of your brain is like the CEO of your entire brain's operation. It handles decision-making, planning, personality, and, you guessed it, **inhibition.** When the frontal lobe is damaged, it throws off your ability to regulate your impulses. Think of it like a power outage in a city's control center. When the lights go out, chaos ensues. Without inhibition, your mind is overrun with impulses you normally would've shut down—like the urge to eat junk food, act recklessly, or say things you don't mean. It's the loss of this internal control that makes life after a brain injury feel chaotic and overwhelming. You find yourself reacting rather than responding, living on autopilot as your impulses take over.

How To Improve Inhibition

The key to improving impulsiveness is through practicing inhibition, meaning that you need to train your brain to pause before acting. When it comes to strengthening your mind and memory, the key once again is about what you do versus what you do not do. Brain cells that you use grow, strengthen, and eventually turn into a network, which is essentially an automated habit. But your brain is a hungry energy organ, this will only take you so far. Because the brain is all about taking the path of least resistance.

So, what do you do? It's very important that you make a gameplan of the thoughts, words, actions, behaviors and habits that you need to **ELIMINATE.**

What a gift it is as a human being that we can make a decision to change our lives! We adapt in response to what we do and what we no longer do! **Inhibition** is the armor that shields you from destructive impulses. Without it, you're a ship without a rudder, driven by cravings and triggers. And it's not just about resisting, it's about taking control of your future self.

Catching The Impulse

To **optimize** your brain power and reclaim control over your life, you have to rebuild your ability to *inhibit*, aka **STOP!** This doesn't happen overnight. Not to beat a dead horse, but science shows that it takes 60-254 days of repeating a behavior for it to become hardwired.

It's like going to the gym. You don't get stronger by lifting the heaviest weight on day one. You get stronger by showing up consistently, lifting what you can, and gradually increasing over time. The same applies to your brain's ability to control impulses.

Start Small and Think Big

Here's a strategy I personally use **DAILY** to catch myself: every time I feel the urge to act impulsively. I will physically stop what I am doing and take a deep breath. That breath creates the pause I need to check myself, assess what's happening, and decide what to do next. This is huge for me in moments when I want to eat something unhealthy, say something reckless, or even give up on my dreams. That one deep breath becomes a gateway to making better choices. **The simple act, of stopping and breathing, puts space between your impulse and your action.** This is where change happens. You might think, "How can a deep breath help me resist my worst habits?" But it does. Breathing resets your nervous system and gives your frontal lobe a chance to re-engage, slowing down that impulse.

You're Not Alone

I know firsthand how difficult this can be. This is simple but definitely not easy! But I'm telling you, **it's sooooo worth it.** The more you work on strengthening your **inhibition**, the more freedom you'll experience in your life. Imagine going a whole day without giving into your past self. Imagine feeling stronger every time you say 'no' to something that doesn't serve you. That's not just possible, **it's *inevitable* if you commit to training your brain.** So, starting today, make it your mission to catch yourself in the moment. Feel that impulse? Take a breath. It's as simple as that. Over time, this small practice will help you rebuild the internal brakes that the concussion stole from you. If you want to really **OPTIMIZE** your brain power, you must get better at catching your **impulses**.

When you strengthen your will power and resolve, you strengthen your **memory**.

Breath Holds And Fasting

Breath holds and fasting are some of the two most powerful tools you can use to strengthen your ability to **inhibit. Quite simply, they are some of the two strongest survival urges we get.** If we can learn to practice resisting these urges, then we can get significantly better at resisting all the other forms of urges. **Breathing** is number one because **without it we will die, very quickly.**

Breathing is the most fundamental function of all life. Without it, our bodies cannot survive. Brain cells begin to die within 3 to 5 minutes without oxygen, leading to irreversible damage around 4 to 6 minutes, and the risk of death significantly increases after 10 minutes. This makes breathing our number one priority for survival.

Why "Breath Control" is so Powerful?

Practicing breath holds can help you build resilience and prepare your mind to cope with stress. When you intentionally hold your breath, you force your body to adapt, promoting mental strength and inhibiting reactive behavior. In a later chapter, I talk about stress management through the principle of "hormesis." There are very few things more effective than holding your breath. It is the most stressful thing to your body. But if you can learn to postpone your breath hold for even a few seconds longer, you can increase your stress tolerance significantly.

Fasting

Fasting is another **primal urge** that can have profound effects on our health and **inhibition**. When you're hungry, your body releases a hormone called ghrelin, which makes you feel the urge to eat. **You know when your stomach growls? That's ghrelin telling you it's time to eat.** But there's another hormone, leptin, that tells your brain when you're full and don't need more food. Even though hunger might feel uncomfortable, taking breaks from eating (like fasting for a few hours) can be really good for your brain and body.

When you fast, your body goes into a kind of clean-up mode called autophagy. It gets rid of old, damaged cells and replaces them with new, healthy ones. This process is not just about weight loss; it's about brain health. Fasting helps reduce inflammation, improve thinking, and even increase the production of brain-derived neurotrophic factor (BDNF), which supports neuron health and growth. The important thing fasting does is help balance your blood sugar (called glucose homeostasis). It lets your body use up the sugar (glucose) it's stored for energy. **When you don't eat for a while, your body starts burning fat instead of sugar.** This helps your body become better at using sugar when it needs to, which is good for keeping things balanced. After fasting for a while, like 12 to 16 hours, your body switches from burning sugar to burning fat. Your liver turns the fat into something called ketones, which your brain can use for energy. When your brain runs on ketones instead of sugar, it works much better! Some people use this idea in a diet called the "Keto Diet," which is full of fat but has very little sugar.

Over time, your brain becomes more efficient at using ketones for energy as your body adapts to low levels of sugar and food. But even though this can be good for your brain in short bursts, it's not something most people should do all the time.

To quickly recap, practicing breathing pauses, breath holds, and fasting are more than just techniques. They are gateways to activate neuroplasticity and profound healing. When your body screams for air or food, challenge yourself to hold on just a little longer. By embracing discomfort, you are priming your neurological and biological self for growth and resilience. You can also apply this principle to other primal urges, such as sexual urges. Practicing self-control over these impulses can strengthen your discipline and enhance your ability to focus on your recovery. By understanding and harnessing these primal urges, you can take significant steps toward brain rescue and overall well-being. Embrace the challenge and empower yourself to become the best version of you!

THE FIFTH STEP IS M FOR MIND GYM:

> *"Your Mind Does Not Get Better By Chance, It Gets Better By Change."*
>
> — JIM ROHN

Why is it universally accepted that if someone commits to the gym, lifting weights, and working out consistently, they'll see impressive physical gains, yet when it comes to the brain, people overlook that it can be "trained" in a similar way? The answer may lie in the visibility of results. With weightlifting, we quickly see our muscles grow and our bodies change, and those physical improvements are undeniable. But brain growth is far less visible, making it easy to underestimate the power and potential of training the brain. Let's make one thing clear: the brain is your body's most vital muscle, the very powerhouse that directs and determines how we function, feel, and flourish.

What Exactly is Mind Gym?

Many people first come across the idea of "mind gym" on social media, where they see me demonstrating exercises that might look quirky or even humorous at first glance. But don't be fooled, these activities are far from being "just for show." **Behind every exercise lies cutting-edge neuroscience designed to stimulate the brain in ways that build brain strength, resilience, and adaptability.** To fully appreciate this, we need to look at the brain's intricate relationship with the body. This brings us to the concept of the homunculus, ever heard of it?

Homunculus... Homuncu-What?

If you're unfamiliar with the term, the homunculus is a representation of the brain that shows us how different parts of the body are mapped in the brain's motor system (movement) and sensory (sensing) areas. It helps us understand how our brain controls and senses our body. On this map, body parts are shown in size according to how much control or feeling they require from the brain. If you look at the picture below, you'll notice that the hands and face are much larger than the other parts. This is because these areas demand lots of fine motor control, and as a result, the brain devotes a substantial amount of 'brain real estate' to manage them. Understanding this map can help explain why moving areas, like the hands, can lead to stronger and more lasting changes in the brain, improving both movement and sensory feedback.

Check out the image of the ugly guy below. Notice how large his hands are relative to the rest of his body.

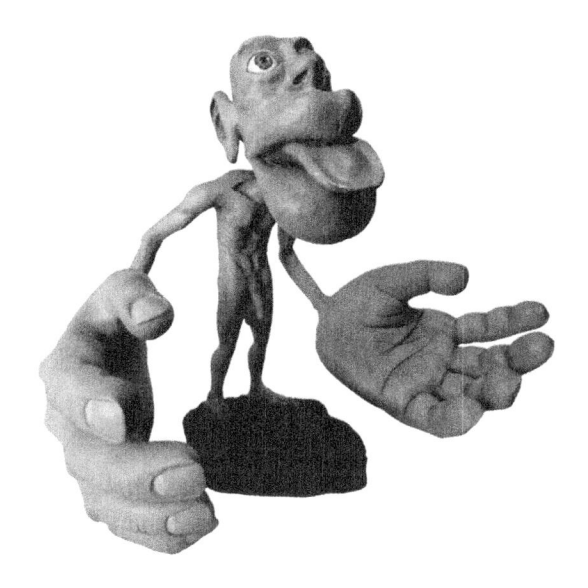

CHAPTER SEVEN: THE FOURTH PILLAR: O IS FOR O.P.T.I.M.I.Z.E • 129

Now check out the diagram below of brain mapping of the motor homunculus for an even better understanding.

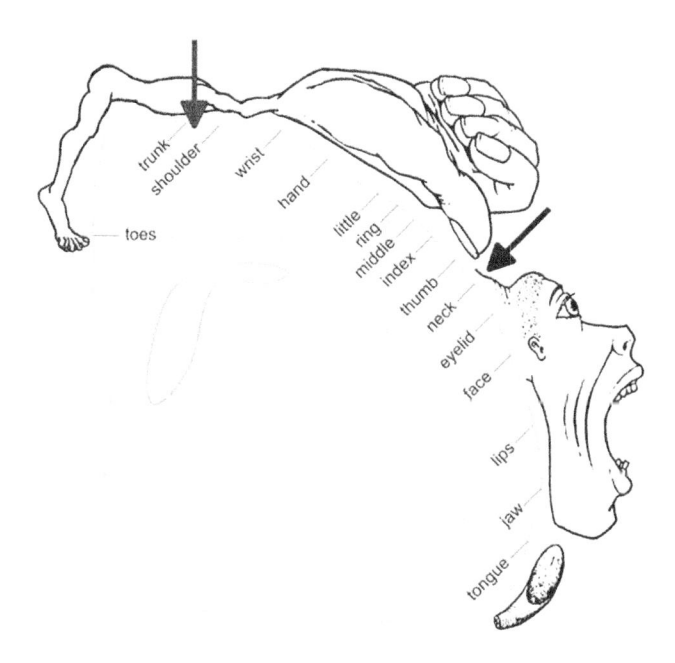

How Mind Gym Aids Brain Injury Recovery

Mind Gym exercises are carefully designed to do more than just get your body moving; they work directly to increase your brain's cognitive load capacity. Cognitive load refers to the amount of mental effort and resources required to perform a task. For people with healthy brains, increasing cognitive load can help build resilience, improve multitasking abilities, and enhance focus. But for those recovering from brain injuries, it serves an even more critical function: it helps rebuild cognitive pathways that may have been damaged or weakened.

Mind gym exercises are in a very real way strengthening your "**neuro muscles**". Consider this. Most gym bros know that skipping leg day, leads to a disproportionate body. They understand that if you only exercise your upper body, it would look weird and leave your lower body way out of balance. The same is true for the brain. Different brain regions serve different functions.

Just as your hands serve a different function than your feet. We don't want to neglect different brain regions. Different mind gym exercises stimulate different brain networks.

Here are 5 Unique Ways Mind Gym Exercises Stimulate the Brain

1. Rewiring the Brain Through Neuroplasticity

After a brain injury, some pathways are wrecked, leaving memory, focus, and processing speed in chaos. But guess what? Neuroplasticity means we can rebuild! Every Mind Gym exercise pushes the brain to forge new connections, retraining areas to take over lost functions and bring back cognitive strength. This isn't just training—it's a rebuild.

2. Building Mental Endurance Gradually

For survivors, the basics feel like heavy lifts. Mind Gym starts simple, then stacks the load, just like a gym routine. You get stronger every day, adding layers of resilience without burnout. Over time, your brain can handle more. Bigger tasks, faster processing, less fatigue.

3. Focus and Attention Control

Focusing, after an injury is a battle. Mind Gym forces focus through simple and controlled movements that demand attention. You retrain that attention muscle until it's sharp and unbreakable. Over time, you regain control and stay locked in when it counts.

4. Boosting Working Memory and Processing Speed

Does your memory feel shot? Exercises like sequencing, counting, and pattern work build your working memory back up. Every movement is a test, and each rep makes your brain faster, ready to recall, react, and crush daily tasks with precision.

5. Reconnecting Body and Brain Coordination

After an injury, your body feels disconnected and clumsy. Mind Gym drills into that brain-body link, syncing up sensory and motor control, bringing back fluidity. This isn't just movement—it's reclaiming coordination and awareness in every move you make.

Take Action Now: Rebuild Your Brain with Mind Gym

Now that you've heard how powerful Mind Gym exercises are, it's now time to experience them firsthand. Don't just read about it; start taking back control of your focus, memory, and resilience today.

Here's how to get started and get 15 Free Mind Gym exercises instantly! Just scan the QR code below or go to www.dr-bro.com/vipbrainrescue to join the VIP Priority list.

This is your invitation to jump in, start strengthening your mind, and feel the results.

THE SIXTH STEP IS I FOR INNER EAR:

> *"The Vestibular System, Located In The Inner Ear, Is So Much More Than A Balance Organ. It Shapes Our Sense Of Movement, Our Ability To Function, And Even Our Emotions."*
>
> — DR. RICHARD DARLINGTON, OTOLARYNGOLOGIST

Alright, listen up! No pun intended. This section is all about optimizing the powerhouse of your inner ear—your vestibular system. **Your vesti-bula what? Yeah, the "vestibular" system!** This term comes from the Latin word **vestibulum**, which means **entrance**. Why do they call it that? Because it's the brain's entry point for auditory and sensory info, keeping you balanced and aware of where you are in space. **Think of your vestibular system as a part of your body's internal GPS System.** It processes info from your inner ear, eyes, and muscles, guiding you through the world and keeping you upright, even when the ground feels wobbly. No more stumbling around like a duck, once you learn how to strengthen this system!

Know the Four Key Players in The Inner Ear

There are **four primary areas** of the inner ear you gotta know, each with its own job:

1. **Saccule**: Activates with up-and-down and vertical movements.

   How it Works: This little guy helps you sense vertical movements—like when you're in an elevator or jumping. It's got fluid and tiny crystals called otoliths. When you move up or down, the fluid shifts, making those crystals move and sending signals to your brain that you're going up or down.

2. **Utricle**: Activates with linear and horizontal movements.

   How It Works: The utricle has your back for side-to-side movements—think walking or running. Like the saccule, it's filled with fluid and otoliths. When you move horizontally, the fluid shifts, sending your brain the signals it needs to know for your position and direction. This keeps you steady while you're on the go.

3. **Horizontal Canal**: Activates with side-to-side and rotational movements.

   How It Works: This is one of three semicircular canals in your inner ear, and it's all about sensing rotational movements. When you turn your head left or right, the fluid inside moves, pushing against tiny hair-like sensors. These send messages to your brain about how your head is turning, keeping your balance on point.

4. **Angular Canals**: Activates with tilting and diagonal movements.

How It Works: The angular canals detect head tilts—like when you nod or lean. There are three of them, each tuned to different tilt directions. As you tilt your head, the fluid moves, activating sensors that let your brain know what's going on. This helps you stay stable, especially when you're reaching or bending.

Why It Matters: Balance and Safety

Here's the deal: **one of the most important jobs of our vestibular system is to prevent us from falling and getting hurt.** Each part works together to keep us balanced. The saccule and utricle signal if we're moving up and down or side to side, helping us adjust our posture to stay upright. The horizontal canal keeps us steady when we turn our heads, ensuring clear vision and quick reactions to dodge obstacles. The angular canals let us know when we tilt our heads, helping coordinate our movements and maintain stability. Overall, your vestibular system is like a balance controller, constantly checking how you move. It keeps you aware of your position, helping you stay on your feet and avoid accidents.

The Connection Between the Vestibular System and Memory

Now, let's talk about how this all connects to **memory**. The vestibular system is vital for both balance and memory. It helps us understand where we are in space, which is crucial for navigating our surroundings. As you move, the vestibular system sends signals to your brain, helping create mental maps of your environment. This connection is super strong with the hippocampus, the part of your brain responsible for forming **memories**. The vestibular system's info aids the hippocampus in remembering routes and locations. [35]

Plus, activities that get you moving, like playing sports or dancing, pump up the vestibular system and boost **memory**. So, taking care of your balance and getting active not only keeps you upright but also sharpens your memory skills. And don't forget about the cerebellum, which means "mini-brain" in Latin. This powerhouse is all about accuracy, balance, and coordination, the A, B, C's of movement. In short, your vestibular system is a key player in how you learn and remember your environment, making it essential for memory rescue. Now get out there and move! Your balance and memory are counting on it!

Take Action: Vestibular System Exercises

Listen up! Let's get your vestibular system firing with these four easy exercises. Each one targets a part of the system to boost your balance and awareness. Let's go!

1. **Saccule (Up and Down):** Reach for the Sky
   - Stand tall. Reach your arms up high like you're trying to touch the ceiling. Then bend down and touch your toes. Repeat 10 times. Feel that stretch! This fires up your saccule.
2. **Utricle (Side to Side):** Side Steps
   - Stand with your feet together. Step right, then bring your left foot to meet it. Now step left and bring your right foot back. Keep going for 1 minute. Simple and effective for your utricle!
3. **Horizontal Canal (Turning):** Head Turns
   - Sit or stand. Keep your body straight and turn your head to the right, then to the left. Do this 10 times. Nice and easy! This gets your horizontal canals working.
4. **Angular Canals (Spinning):** Kid's Circle Spins
   - Stand with feet shoulder-width apart. Now, start spinning in a circle like a kid! Do this nice and easy for 30 seconds, then switch directions with CARE! This playful movement stimulates your angular canals and helps with balance.

Major key: Do these exercises with care. If you feel dizzy, nauseous, or unbalanced, slow down. Change your pace, frequency, and intensity. Go as slow as you need to. It's all about progress, not perfection or competition.

Get after it! Do these exercises a minimum of 1-2 times a week to sharpen your balance and memory. Stay consistent, and watch your skills improve!

THE SEVENTH STEP IS Z FOR ZERO DISTRACTIONS:

> *"In the Age of Distraction, Focusing On One Thing is a Superpower."*
>
> — JAMES CLEAR

Listen up! If you want to rise above the noise in this chaotic world, you need to embrace the concept of Zero Distractions. In 2025, we are living in a fast-paced world, where notifications and interruptions lurk around every corner. The ability to focus deeply on a single task is the most important thing you can do to set yourself apart from the rest of the world.

Let me tell you something: productivity isn't about how much work you can grind away. It's about the quality of what you produce.

When you **FOCUS** on only one activity at a time your productivity will **SKYROCKET. FOCUS IS KEY!** In a world that glorifies busy work, you need to flip the script. When you commit to deep focus, you'll not only maximize your productivity you will maximize your brain power.

The Neuroscience Of Focus & Memory

Here's the scoop on focus: your brain is like a well-organized team, with each part playing a unique role to help you concentrate, make decisions, and stay on track. Focus is like a symphony, with different brain regions and neurotransmitters playing harmoniously to help you concentrate, make decisions, and excel.

- **Prefrontal Cortex**: The strategic coach guiding your decision-making and keeping you on task.
- **Anterior Cingulate Cortex**: Your internal motivator, pushing you through challenges.
- **Parietal Lobe**: The spatial awareness expert, ensuring you stay grounded in your environment.
- **Thalamus**: The gatekeeper, filtering distractions to keep your focus razor-sharp.
- **Basal Ganglia**: The taskmaster, ensuring you stay consistent and on track.
- **Amygdala**: The emotional powerhouse, influencing whether your feelings enhance or hinder focus.
- **Hippocampus**: Your memory vault, holding onto key information.
- **Insula**: The bridge between feelings and attention, helping you prioritize.
- **Cerebellum**: The precision engineer, fine-tuning actions for optimal results.

Wow, there's a lot going on behind the scenes, right?

Studies from the University of California show that office workers are typically interrupted every 11 minutes, yet it takes 25 minutes for them to refocus. [36] Imagine the compounding effect of reducing these interruptions!

When you focus with **Zero Distractions,** you're not just finishing today's to-do list: you're getting closer to your dreams. By focusing deeply, you'll make consistent progress on what truly matters.

Every time you get distracted, your brain is forced to switch to something else, and that wastes a lot of precious energy. This is called 'context switching,' and it can take a really long time to fully get your brain back to where it was, making it a silent productivity killer. [37]

Many people still think multitasking is productive, but research shows it reduces efficiency by up to 40%. [38] Real productivity comes from doing one thing at a time with undivided attention.

Multi-tasking and task-switching can be helpful to brain health and survival, but not when it comes to focusing and doing your best work.

If you reduce distractions and work on one thing at a time, you'll see your productivity and focus grow. You'll build momentum, get closer to sharpening your **memory** and achieving your goals.

So, take charge of your time. Focus on one task, get rid of as many interruptions as possible, and watch how you move toward the life you've always wanted. Focusing is your superpower, so use it to your advantage!

T.O.T. 90 For Max Productivity

1. Schedule It

- Set a specific time for your focused work session. Treat it like an important meeting or appointment. Put it in your calendar, set a reminder, and commit to showing up. Having a clear time frame helps ensure that you're not rushing or procrastinating.

2. Clear the Space

- Eliminate all distractions and noises from your environment before you start. Put your phone in another room, close all unnecessary tabs or apps, tidy up your physical workspace. Make sure if you have kids that they don't distract you either. Put on noise-canceling headphones for an added effect.

3. Do It, Refocus Constantly

- Start your task and commit to staying focused for the full 90 minutes, as much as you possibly can. When distractions or stray thoughts pop up (and they will), gently refocus your mind back to the task. Acknowledge the distraction but don't engage with it. The key is to stay persistent and keep returning your attention to the work.

4. Reward Yourself

- Once your 90-minute focus session is complete, give yourself a reward. It could be a short break, a treat, or something you enjoy. This not only gives you a mental reset but also reinforces the habit of staying focused, making it more likely you'll repeat it the next time.

This strategy will help skyrocket your productivity and will put you ahead of 95% of the population that is constantly distracted. Remember, practice makes progress, then permanent.

THE EIGHTH STEP IS E FOR EMOTIONS:

> *"The Emotion That Can Break Your Heart is Sometimes the Very One That Heals it."*
>
> — NICHOLAS SPARKS

E-MOTIONS (ENERGY-IN-MOTION) are among the most powerful forces in your recovery and life. All the effort to **OPTIMIZE** your brain will be meaningless if you don't intently focus on creating positive emotions. Why? Because the quality of your recovery, your memory, your focus, and ultimately your life is a direct reflection of the quality of your emotions.

Your Emotional Home

Think about your day-to-day life. Have you noticed that certain **emotions** seem to dominate no matter what happens? The fact is, most of us experience the same 5 or 6 core emotions regularly, regardless of the external circumstances. Maybe it's frustration when you forget where you put **your stuff** at a coffee shop or the anxiety that pills up when you can't focus at work. This is like your emotional **"default setting"** or personal home base. No matter how far you stray, whether experiencing a fleeting moment of joy or a surge of anger, you always seem to return to these familiar **emotional states.** These feelings form your emotional home. They are the set of emotions you naturally return to day by day. **No matter** how far you go away, you will **always** find your emotional home. The exciting truth is that your emotional home doesn't have to be permanent. It can be **redesigned**, just like you might renovate your physical home. By understanding and working with your emotions, you can create a more stable, positive foundation that supports your **healing** and **empowers** your **recovery** journey.

The Purpose of Negative Emotions

Think of **emotions** as neither **negative or positive**; they just are. Even the emotions that feel the most terrifying and brutal serve an underlying purpose. **Fear** and **anxiety**, for example, are like your brain's internal **alarm system**, sharpening your focus to potential threats. Even frustration can be a force that propels you to **change** things you don't like in your life.

But **living** in these emotions for **too long** can become **draining**, like trying to **swim** in **stormy waters** for days on end. That's why it's **important** to foster **balance** by actively **creating** emotions like **gratitude, hope, and joy**, which help calm your nervous system and allow your brain to **heal.**

Riding the Emotional Waves

Emotions are like **waves** in the ocean that **come and go**. They are **natural, ever-changing, and unavoidable**. Sometimes, the waves are **calm**, coming **gently** at your feet, while others are **violent and turbulent, crashing** into you with an **intensity** that can leave you gasping for air.

Imagine you're out in the ocean of your mind. The **waves** represent your **emotions**: frustration. sadness, anxiety, and even joy. You can't stop these waves from forming, and you sure as hell **can't control** their size or timing. But you can **learn** how to **navigate** them, to ride them, rather than trying to fight against them.

When the **water** is choppy, your first instinct may be to **resist**. But trying to fight the waves is exhausting and futile. **Throwing rocks** at the ocean and the ocean will laugh at you. It will only pull you deeper into the tide. Instead, you can choose to **acknowledge** the waves as they are and choose to focus on using them to your **advantage**.

Even the most skilled surfers fall sometimes. There will be moments when an **emotional wave** feels too big and will drag you under. That's okay. The **key** is to **refocus, take a deep breath,** and get back on your board. Each time you **practice**, you will become **stronger, more courageous,** and more skilled at navigating the highs and lows.

Emotions and Your Healing

Here's the fascinating part: the way you handle these emotional waves has a **direct impact** on your brain's ability to heal itself. Positive emotions like **gratitude** and **love** trigger the release of neurotransmitters such as **dopamine, serotonin, and oxytocin,** which enhance **neuroplasticity**. By cultivating positive emotional waves and learning to gracefully navigate the stormy ones, you're not only improving your quality of life but actively rewiring your brain to support focus, memory, and resilience.

Become the Master Surfer in Three Steps

Learning to ride the emotional waves doesn't mean avoiding or suppressing them. In fact, suppression often makes the waves stronger and more unpredictable. It's like trying to hold a beach ball underwater, it will eventually burst back up with force.

Instead, embrace the waves with curiosity and acceptance. When you feel a surge of frustration, pause and ask yourself: *What is this emotion trying to tell me?* By observing rather than reacting, you allow the wave to pass naturally.

Three Practical Strategies To Master Emotional Surfing:

1. **Practice Awareness:** Check in with yourself throughout the day. Close your eyes and ask, "What am I feeling right now?" Naming the emotion without judgment helps you step back and understand it.
2. **Anchor Yourself:** When the waves feel overwhelming, ground yourself with a calming practice, such as deep breathing or visualization. Imagine you're on a surfboard, staying steady as the water moves beneath you.
3. **Cultivate Calming Waves:** Actively create emotions like gratitude, hope, and joy. These emotions act like gentle tides, soothing the nervous system and creating the optimal environment for your brain to heal.

Referring back to the main point. Everyone reading this has the freedom to channel all of your emotions into positive action.

Take the suggestions, however you will, but these are a bit general but generally good suggestions.

Depressed about your situation? Change it.

Mad? Harness your anger enough to force change.

Angry about the economy? Go to the gym.

Everyone of your emotions can be channeled into positive action in the world.

Every emotion is simply fuel to propel you to the highest level of success.

Therefore, there are no real BAD emotions.

Only bad use of emotions.

Remember, becoming a master surfer takes practice. Some days, the ocean will feel calm and manageable. On other days, it may feel wild and relentless. But each time you ride a wave, you're building strength, balance, and confidence, key skills for reclaiming your brain's potential and creating the life you deserve.

CHAPTER EIGHT: THE FIFTH PILLAR: U IS FOR U.N.L.E.A.S.H

THE FIRST STEP IS U FOR UNCONSCIOUS BRAIN:

Did you know your unconscious brain controls 95% of your thoughts, behaviors, and actions? It's like the invisible driver steering your life. **Your unconscious brain is incredibly powerful.** It's where your automatic behaviors live, like how you instinctively know how to walk, breathe, or even react without thinking about it. Your conscious brain is what you use to define, articulate, and set goals. But it's your unconscious mind that follows through with all the hundreds of millions of actions necessary to achieve those goals. To help you understand it's incredible power, I am going to source from the book, "The Answer" By John Assaraf and Murray Smith.

- Conscious impulse travels at 120-140 mph. Nonconscious impulses travel at speeds of more than 100,000 mph, or 800 times faster than conscious impulses.
- The conscious brain processes about 2,000 bits of information per second. The nonconscious brain processes about 400,000,000,000 (four hundred billion) bits of information per second.

- **The conscious brain operates with a very short-term memory span. Generally limited to about twenty seconds. The nonconscious brain remembers everything it experiences forever.** [39]

Top tier neuroscientists like Dr. Andrew Huberman have confirmed this is no longer just a **FEEL-GOOD THEORY**. It's backed by hard science.

For someone like you, recovering from a brain injury, understanding and tapping into your unconscious brain is a game-changer. Why? Because it's the key to creating new neural connections and rewiring your brain for lasting healing. Focused mental practices, like visualization, can increase the speed of recovery and even help your brain create stronger pathways to rebuild damaged areas. By learning how to harness the power of your unconscious mind, you can train it to focus on healing and resilience. **Techniques like mindfulness, positive affirmations, or specific guided exercises can help shift your brain's automatic responses from stress or frustration to calmness and hope.** This can reduce stress hormones, improve sleep, and give your brain the space it needs to heal. Mastering this part of your mind doesn't just help you recover; it sets you up for long-term success. It gives you the tools to overcome setbacks, take control of your thoughts, and build a future that's even stronger than before. Recovery starts with belief, and belief starts in your unconscious brain.

5 Stages Of Learning

Learning any new skill, behavior, or habit involves progressing through **five distinct stages.** Understanding where you are in this journey will help you overcome doubt and frustration. As we've discussed, **learning** new information sparks new ideas. New ideas lead to experiences, which create stronger and more vivid **memories.** Let's apply these ideas to the brain health recovery process.

Stronger more robust **memories** enhance brain health, and better brain health leads to a better life!

1. Uninformed Optimism (Unconscious Incompetence)

At this stage, you simply **don't know what you don't know.** You are unaware of how much you need to learn or how challenging the road to recovery will be. Ignorance can feel blissful, and you may be overconfident, fueled by optimism and the hope of a quick fix.

Typical thoughts and feelings:

- "I'll be back to normal in no time. How hard can this really be?"
- "I've always been a fast learner. This shouldn't take long."
- "I'll just follow a few tips I found online, and I'll be good as new."

At this point, the lack of awareness creates a sense of overconfidence. You might eagerly dive into recovery plans without fully understanding the complexities of brain rehabilitation.

2. Informed Pessimism (Conscious Incompetence)

This is when reality starts to set in. You become hightly aware of your limitations and the amount of effort required for progress. This stage can be disheartening as the excitement fades, and self-doubt begins to creep in.

Typical thoughts and feelings:

- "This is way harder than I expected. Why isn't my brain responding faster?"
- "I thought I'd feel better by now. Maybe I'll never get back to where I was."
- "Every step forward feels like two steps back. Why can't I just think clearly?"

During this stage, frustration builds as you realize recovery isn't linear. This awareness can trigger fear, anger, or even hopelessness, but it's also the first sign of growth.

3. Valley of Despair (The Turning Point)

This isn't a traditional stage of competence but a critical emotional stage in recovery. It's the moment when progress feels stagnant, and the gap between effort and results seems insurmountable. Many survivors are tempted to quit here, but this is also where breakthroughs often begin.

Typical thoughts and feelings:

- "Why am I even trying? It feels like I'll never get better."
- "I'm exhausted, and nothing seems to be working. Maybe this is just my new normal."
- "I've done everything they told me to do, but I still feel stuck."

While it's the darkest point, the Valley of Despair is also the turning point. If you can persevere, often with support and guidance, you'll begin to see incremental but meaningful improvements. Please don't give up when you reach this stage, even though it's hard.

4. Informed Optimism (Conscious Competence)

You've pushed through the despair and are now seeing real progress. You understand what works for your brain and are building skills that require effort but are yielding results. Confidence begins to return, and you're more in tune with your recovery process.

Typical thoughts and feelings:

- "Finally, I'm starting to feel like myself again."
- "This is hard work, but it's paying off. I'm stronger than I thought."
- "I'm not 100% yet, but I can see the path forward."

This stage feels rewarding as the efforts you've invested start to translate into tangible results. Lots of small victories to fuel your determination to keep moving forward.

5. Success and Fulfillment (Unconscious Competence)

Now you've reached mastery in certain aspects of your recovery. The skills and habits you've built have become second nature, allowing you to function effectively without overthinking each step. You feel a sense of accomplishment and renewed confidence.

Typical thoughts and feelings:

- "I'm finally thriving, not just surviving."
- "I can't believe how far I've come. I never thought I'd get here."
- "Recovery wasn't just about healing my brain; it taught me how resilient I truly am."

This stage is about celebrating your progress while remaining mindful that recovery is an ongoing journey. At this stage, you've reached mastery! The skill or habit has become second nature, you do it effortlessly and instinctively, like Michael Jordan nailing a free throw or Tiger Woods hitting a perfect swing. However, this mastery didn't happen overnight. It was the result of consistent, deliberate practice over time.

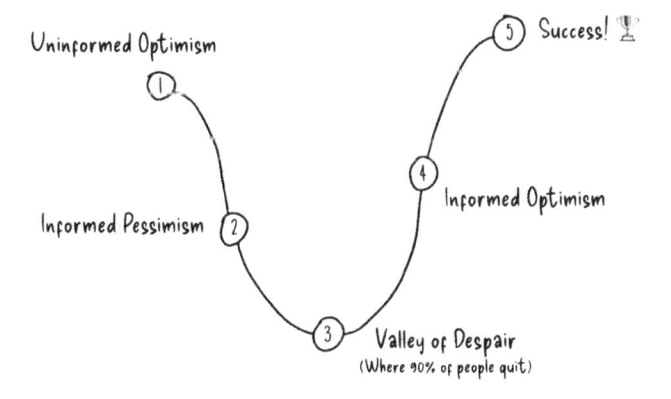

Uninformed Optimism (1) → Informed Pessimism (2) → Valley of Despair (3) (Where 90% of people quit) → Informed Optimism (4) → Success! (5)

ACTION STEP!

- **S.M.A.R.T. GOALS**- **S**pecific (Clearly Define Your Goal), **M**easurable (Track your progress), **A**chievable (Set goals you can realistically accomplish), **R**elevant (Your goal should align with your overall vision and purpose), **T**ime (Give Yourself a Deadline to create urgency in your mind)

TAKE ACTION TOWARDS A BETTER MEMORY TODAY in Three Simple Steps!

Step 1: Write down one S.M.A.R.T Goal in the form of an "I WANT" statement for a SPECIFIC area of your life you want to improve. Example: I want to lose 5 pounds by December 31st.

Step 2: Write down THREE Strategies to increase the chances of you realistically being able to achieve that goal.

Examples

Strategy (A) Walk for 10 minutes every morning to burn calories.

Strategy (B) Track and reduce daily calorie intake by 10% using the MyfitnessPal app.

Strategy (C): Drink 128 FL ounces of water daily to hydrate the body and reduce hunger pains.

STEP 3: Repeat 5-7 days a week until you accomplish your goal.

(Always remember WHY you are doing the goal in the first place!

Example: I am losing weight and moving more because it will improve my memory!)

THE SECOND STEP IS <u>N</u> FOR NERVE:

> *"You Got Some Real Nerve About You, Don't You Pal?!"*
>
> — DR. BRODY :)

Did you know there are an estimated 7 trillion nerves in the human body? Nerve signals can travel as fast as 200 miles per hour (about 320 kilometers per hour), enabling quick reflexes and rapid muscle movement.

Have you ever been to Vegas? No, I am not talking about the place where you go to party, do drugs, and look for late-night adventure. **Get your mind out of the gutter!**

I'm talking about the largest nerve in the human body. **The Vagus nerve, 10th cranial nerve, or cranial nerve x, is the longest cranial nerve in the body**, running from the brainstem down to the colon, branching throughout vital organs like the heart, lungs, and digestive tract. But the Vagus nerve isn't just a simple connection from brain to body; it's part of a sophisticated network that communicates signals from your organs back to your brain, helping the brain to regulate bodily functions based on real-time feedback.

The Vagus nerve alone has around **80,000** to **100,000** fibers helping to regulate heart rate, digestion, and even emotional stability.

The Vagus nerve is like a superhighway with two main lanes, each going in different directions and doing different jobs in the body and mind. These two lanes are called the **dorsal vagal pathway and the ventral vagal pathway.**

The **dorsal vagal pathway** is the body's "shutdown" button, connecting to the oldest, most basic parts of our nervous system—kind of like the "reptile brain" that all animals have.

The term Dorsal is derived from the Latin word "dorsalis", which means "of the back."

When this pathway is engaged, it controls things like resting, digesting food, and helping the body relax and save energy. But, when life throws something really intense or scary at you, this pathway can go into full shutdown mode, almost like hitting a power-off button. When that happens, you might feel numb, detached, or even "frozen" to protect your body from too much stress. So, in regular times, the dorsal vagal pathway helps the body chill and recharge, but in tough times, it can make us shut down to handle the overload.

The **ventral vagal pathway** is like your body's "social superhero." It connects to the brain areas that help us communicate, connect, and stay focused. **Ventral** comes from the Latin word **"ventralis,"** meaning "of the belly" referring to the front or belly side of an organism.

Dr. Stephen Porges the founder of Polyvagal theory calls the ventral pathway the "social engagement system." When this pathway is working, it sends messages to your heart and lungs, keeping you calm but alert—perfect for clear thinking and making memories.

Unlike the dorsal pathway, which can make you shut down, the ventral vagal pathway helps you stay open and engaged with the world around you. It's what allows you to handle social situations, control your emotions, and really connect with other people. When this pathway is active, you're ready to interact, learn, and grow!

The Vagus nerve is unique because it doesn't operate as a simple one-way street. Two main areas of the vagus nerve serve different functions is our body and mind.

Let's Get A Little Nervy

Activating the ventral vagus nerve taps into the body's power to regulate bodily systems, which can impact everything from heart rate and inflammation to emotional stability and cognitive function. Let's break down some of the key benefits of brain injury recovery.

1. Reduces Inflammation

- Activates anti-inflammatory brain pathways. This is particularly beneficial for brain injury survivors, as inflammation in the brain can exacerbate symptoms and delay recovery.

2. Regulates the Nervous System

- Helps shift the body out of the "fight-or-flight" state (sympathetic dominance) and into a "rest-and-digest" state, promoting healing and reducing stress.

3. Promotes Emotional Regulation.

- Can reduce symptoms of anxiety, depression, and mood swings, by influencing brain areas like the prefrontal cortex and the amygdala.

4. Better Sleep Quality

- Head injuries often disrupt sleep patterns. Activating the vagus nerve can help restore balance to the nervous system, improving sleep duration and quality.

5. Enhances Cognitive Functioning

- Vagus nerve stimulation has been shown to improve attention, memory and executive function, which are commonly impaired in brain injury survivors.

5 Natural Ways to Stimulate the Vagus Nerve

1. Gargling, Humming, Singing.

Reduces stress and enhances relaxation. Activates throat muscles, promoting parasympathetic response.

2. Extended Exhalations.

Long exhales trigger the parasympathetic system. Promotes relaxation and lowers heart rate

3. Deep Breathing.

Deep breaths stimulate the vagus nerve via the diaphragm. It calms the nervous system and reduces stress. [40]

4. Cold Therapy.

Cold exposure activates the vagus nerve and calms the fight-or-flight response. Reduces stress and strengthens the immune system

5. Using Vagus Nerve Stimulators (e.g., Truvaga)

Electrical pulses directly stimulate the vagus nerve. Rapidly reduces anxiety and improves heart rate variability.

At the time of the writing, I am not affiliated with the company Truvaga, but I have received a trial of their product, and it has been extremely effective and amazing in reducing my stress levels over the last month while writing this book. My sleep has improved, and the best part is you only need to use the product for four minutes a day for amazing results! Once in the morning and once at night. I like to be my own science experiment. Just a heads up!

THE THIRD STEP IS L FOR LYMPHATICS:

> *"Your Lymphatic System Is The River Of Life, Flowing Through You To Nourish, Protect, And Cleanse Your Cells."*
>
> — DR. BRUCE BERKOWSKY

The **lymphatic system** is perhaps the most overlooked system in the entire human body. It plays a huge role in keeping us healthy. Think of it as the **body's drainage system**, responsible for removing toxins, waste, and other harmful stuff. Without it, our immune system wouldn't work well, and we'd be more likely to get sick. However, many people don't realize how important it is to take care of this system, even though it helps with things like balancing fluids, detoxifying the body, and keeping our immune system strong.

I had the opportunity to talk to **Dr. Perry Nickelston, known as "The Lymph Doc"** from Stop Chasing Pain. He explained that the lymphatic system is like a plumbing system in your house. **Every major lymph node in your body is like a little toilet or drain. When these drains work properly, they flush out the bad stuff. But when they get blocked or clogged, it's like having a backed-up drain in your house**—it causes problems and makes you feel sick.

A brain injury can make this even worse. The brain has its own system, called the glymphatic system, which works like the lymphatic system but for your brain. It clears away waste, especially while you sleep. After a brain injury, this system doesn't work as well, causing toxins to build up and slowing down healing. That's why helping the lymphatic system do its job is so important—it can reduce swelling, get rid of toxins, and help your brain recover faster.

Action Step: Start with Dr. Perry's Big 6 Tm Lymph Reset

To keep your lymphatic system flowing properly, Dr. Perry recommends starting with six key areas in your body that often get blocked. These are simple, quick movements that help get your lymph fluid moving. Here's what to do:

1. **Collarbone**: Gently rub the area just below your collarbones. Rub your hand slowly in a circular direction 10 times. After that, do ten light taps. Repeat on the other side.
2. **Upper Neck:** Find the next spot on the side of the neck, below the lobe of the ear where the largest lymph node in the neck sits. It may feel a little tender. Now simultaneously rub both spots gently 10 times in a circle motion, then lightly tap 10 times.
3. **Pectoral/Axillary** Find the spot at the shoulder joint where the pectoral muscle meets your deltoid, called the axillary region. Put your hand over that region and turn your arm out a little bit. Rub ten times and tap ten times. Then repeat on the other side.
4. **Abdominal/Navel.** Put one hand over the navel and one hand above. Rub in circles 10 times. Then lightly tap 10 times.
5. **Inguinal (Groin)** This spot is at the crease of the groin. Simultaneously rub in circles on both sides for 10, then lightly tap for 10.
6. **Popliteal (Behind the Knees)**: Gently rub in circles behind your knees for 10. Then tap for ten.
7. **Now do some Self-Rebounding.** Jump up and down using your calf muscles. Lightly bounce. Then shake out your arms at the same time. Do that for 30 seconds to one minute.

THE FOURTH STEP IS E FOR EES (ENERGY ENHANCEMENT SYSTEM):

> *"Energy Cannot Be Created Or Destroyed, It Can Only Be Changed From One Form To Another."*
>
> — ALBERT EINSTEIN

Unleash A New Era of Wellness

The Energy Enhancement System (EESystem) combines the science of body, mind, spirit, to unleash your full potential, fostering peak performance and unlocking higher levels of health, consciousness, and self-actualization. I call it "consciousness medicine" in how it changes your consciousness. This system generates special energy fields, like "scalar waves," that support cell regeneration, boost circulation, strengthen immune function, and reduce inflammation. It offers relief from pain, aids detoxification, elevates mood, and balances brain hemispheres, optimizing meditation and sleep. Additionally, EESystem enhances memory, focus, and cognitive clarity by energizing cell membranes, activating mitochondria, and promoting neuroplasticity for optimal brain function.

The Energy Enhancement System

Dr. Sandra Rose Michael developed a groundbreaking healing technology that many consider to be more advanced than "Med Bed Technology." First introduced in 1997, the system uses custom-calibrated computers to generate morphogenic energy fields. By combining quantum physics and genetic amplification, the EESystem enables cellular regeneration and healing from within, empowering users to unleash their body's natural potential by increasing the voltage of your cells.[41] Recognized globally at medical and scientific conferences, it continues to revolutionize approaches to wellness.

Transformative Benefits Reported by Users

Individual experiences vary, but users frequently report:

- Enhanced memory, focus, and cognitive clarity
- Profound calmness, relaxation, and emotional harmony
- Natural healing and accelerated rejuvenation
- Heightened energy and vitality
- Relief from depression and brain fog
- Greater emotional freedom and mental flexibility
- Reduced attachment to past traumas
- Improved mindfulness and presence
- Better responses to stressors and life's challenges
- Peak physical and mental performance

The Energy Enhancement System can also help people recover quickly after surgery, improve their blood health, detoxify, and live in a more empowered, authentic way. It's like a "reset" for your body and mind, making you feel more balanced and clear-headed. Many users describe it as calming, reducing stress and helping them focus better. If you've had trouble with memory, it can be life-changing. People often report having sharper memory, better focus, and feeling more energized, which helps them think more clearly and feel more in control of their lives. This "frequency bath" offers a chance for your body and mind to reconnect and perform at their best.

I personally have noticed huge changes in my own health and quantifiable improvements in my sleep using the Oura ring. Not only that, but every time I go to the ESS system I feel much more energy and libido with my wife. Haha. TMI, I know...

Take Action Find A Center Near You

Simply go to **www.eesystem.com/center-locater** and search for a center close to you. Book a session and go! I 100% guarantee you won't regret it. I have no affiliations with any of the EES system companies or centers. Only the desire to help others get better as soon as possible.

THE FIFTH STEP IS A FOR ATTENTION

> *"The Universe responds to the vibrational frequency of your attention."*
>
> — DEEPAK CHOPRA

Did you know that our attention is the largest gateway to **memory enhancement**? It acts like a spotlight, illuminating the things you deem important while leaving the rest in the shadows. **Let me let you in on a very important secret. Where attention flows, blood flow goes.** [42] When you focus your attention on a particular task or idea, your brain channels resources to that area, enhancing both mental clarity and retention. In other words, where you put your attention is where you put your energy. **What you put your ATTENTION on expands and multiples!** So be very careful about what you choose to focus on. And trust me, this is a choice. Harnessing attention is crucial for sharpening your memory, especially when facing the challenges of brain fog or memory lapses.

Let me prove this to you. **Think about a time when you desired something deeply**—perhaps a specific car like a red Jeep. Before you wanted one, you probably noticed very few red Jeeps on the road. Now that you have the means to buy one, they have become relevant, and it seems as if they're popping up everywhere!

But why is that? The truth is, those red Jeeps were always there, parked in driveways or cruising by. **The difference lies in your focus.** Previously, your thalamus was busy generalizing, filtering, and deleting what it deemed irrelevant. However, now that owning a red Jeep is significant to you, your **Reticular Activating System** (RAS) kicks in, spotlighting those vehicles in your environment. RAS is the neuroscientific term for a complex network of neurons located in the brainstem that plays a crucial role in regulating wakefulness, attention, and the filtering of sensory information to prioritize what we perceive as most important. [43]

It actively seeks out what matters to you, enhancing your awareness and memory of those instances. Every day, we are bombarded with millions of pieces of information—from social media notifications to conversations happening around us. Our brains constantly filter out the noise to prevent us from feeling overwhelmed. But when we choose to focus on specific topics, emotions, or experiences, we train our brains to recognize patterns and make connections.

To make your attention work for you, make sure to focus on what you want to remember or to get better at. For example, if you want to remember someone's name, pay special extra attention when you meet them. Try to picture their name in your mind, link it to something memorable, and say it to yourself. The more you practice, the stronger your brain will get at remembering. By choosing where you focus, you can shape what you notice and improve your memory.

In essence, you're not just observing the world around you—you're actively shaping your reality by what you choose to pay attention to.

Now, let's dive deeper into actionable strategy that will help you channel your focus effectively, so you can sharpen your memory and reclaim your mental clarity!

Take Massive Action NOW! Candle Focus Drill

Light a candle. **For the next 10 minutes, lock your eyes on that flame.** Watch it flicker—feel your focus tighten. When distractions hit (and they will), don't fight them—acknowledge and snap your attention back. Every time you do, you're sharpening your mind and building an unbreakable focus. This exercise engages the executive network of your brain, enhancing focus, mental clarity, and visual processing. **Repeat 3-5 times weekly.**

THE SIXTH STEP IS S FOR SUPER LEARNING:

> *An Investment In Knowledge Always Pays The Best Interest."*
>
> — BENJAMIN FRANKLIN

We're not just talking about learning here; we're talking about **Super-learning!** Do you want a great **memory**? Then you've got to level up the way you process and retain information, period. Let me break it down for you in a way you'll understand. **Super learning is about locking in as much new knowledge as you can, as fast as you can, so that it sticks with you and elevates your game.** This isn't just some random gimmick; it's a way to rewire your brain for greatness. This is about learning and retaining as much information as possible!

So, what's the plan? We're going to engage the brain in a multi-faceted way.

Pro-Tip: Did you know that when you read, listen, and write, you activate different areas of your brain? Your brain has different regions that light up when you take in information through different modes. When you read, you're stimulating your visual cortex; when you listen, you're firing up the auditory cortex; and when you write, you're engaging the motor and prefrontal cortex. You've got to tap into all these areas to get the full experience.

Therefore, if you make sure to learn in these three dynamic ways, you are strengthening different networks of the brain in a holistic way. **This will allow you to learn at a faster rate than you ever thought possible while simultaneously increasing the amount of info that you retain!**

I know it's been mentioned so many damn times in the book already but it's true! Always consider your brain to be like a mental muscle. You don't just do one exercise to build your body; you hit the weights from every angle to build balanced strength. The same goes for Super-learning. Reading is like doing your bench presses, hitting the visual cortex hard. Listening is like adding in core exercises, targeting that auditory cortex, and laying a strong foundation. Writing is like doing squats; it hits deep. It's where things come together, and you level up. It's like cross-training for your mind!

Let me ask you a few hard questions because if I don't ask you these questions, who will? How badly do you really want to improve? How committed are you to making this change? Because if you're not willing to go all in on this, you might as well stay in that same place you've been stuck in for years. But if you're ready to step up, to do the work, and to change how you approach learning, then we can make some serious progress. When you just read something, you're getting maybe 10-20% of the full benefit. It's like trying to work out only one side of your body. But when you combine reading, listening, and writing, you're getting a synergy effect. The act of reading brings the concepts to life visually. Your eyes track the words, and your brain starts processing the information in real-time, creating an internal dialogue. Then, when you listen to the same information or someone else explaining it, you reinforce what you've read. The auditory cortex engages as you activate Wernicke's area (language processing) and suddenly, the concepts go from static to dynamic. Finally, when you write down what you've learned, you're not just passively processing the information anymore. You're taking an active role in reshaping the structure of your brain, engaging motor cortex, and Broca's area (language production) and enhancing your brain's ability to retain that info long-term.

THE SEVENTH STEP IS H IS FOR HORMESIS!!!:

> *"Out Of This Delicate Balance Of Tension And Release, Struggle And Rest, We Build Resilience."*
>
> — DAVID GOGGINS

Just like anything else in life, too much or too little of anything can be detrimental to our health. Take water, for example. If you have little water, you will suffer from dehydration, but if you have too much, you will have water poisoning and can eventually drown. The same goes for stress. Too little can debilitate you, and too much can cause a heart attack. The **hormesis principle**, often referred to as the **hormesis effect**, revolves around understanding stress thresholds and their impact on our health and performance. At its core, hormesis teaches us that not all stress is harmful—in fact, the right kind of stress can be incredibly beneficial. It's about finding that sweet spot in the amount or dosage in our lives.

When we talk about stress, it's essential to differentiate between **eustress (positive stress)** and **distress (negative stress)**. Eustress is the type of stress that motivates us, pushes us to grow, and enhances our overall well-being. This positive stress is vital for our bodies and minds to thrive. Negative stress is toxic and cause our bodies to get extremely sick. Consider this: if a person doesn't engage in any physical activity, they experience too little stress on their muscles. Over time, this lack of stress leads to muscle weakening and atrophy, essentially, their muscles deteriorate because they're not being used. This example highlights how a certain amount of physical stress is necessary to maintain muscle strength, endurance, and overall physical health.

Similarly, in the realm of brain health, a lack of mental challenges, whether through learning new skills, solving puzzles, or engaging in stimulating conversations, can lead to cognitive decline and memory loss. Our brains need the right amount of stress to forge new neural connections and promote neuroplasticity, which is crucial for recovery from brain injuries and maintaining cognitive function as we age.

In essence, the hormesis principle teaches us that stress, when applied correctly, acts as a catalyst for growth and recovery. It encourages our bodies and brains to adapt and strengthen in the face of challenges. However, the key lies in moderation. Too much stress of any form can overwhelm our systems, leading to negative health effects.

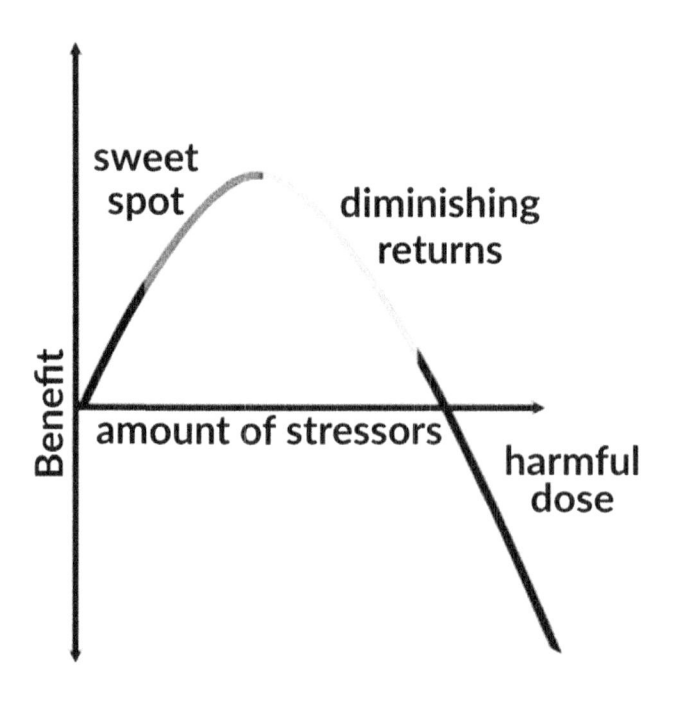

(Graph: Benefit vs. amount of stressors, showing "sweet spot", "diminishing returns", and "harmful dose")

Understanding the HPA Axis

Now, let's discuss the HPA axis, which stands for the hypothalamic-pituitary-adrenal axis. This is a complex set of interactions between three key glands: the hypothalamus, the pituitary gland, and the adrenal glands. Together, they play a crucial role in how our body responds to stress and why so many people have adrenal fatigue and burnout.

1. **Hypothalamus:** This gland is located deep in the limbic brain and detects stress. When it senses stress, it releases a hormone called corticotropin-releasing hormone (CRH).
2. **Pituitary Gland:** In response to CRH, the pituitary gland releases adrenocorticotropic hormone (ACTH) into the bloodstream.
3. **Adrenal Glands:** ACTH signals the adrenal glands (located on top of your kidneys) to produce cortisol, a hormone that helps your body manage stress.

Cortisol is essential for many bodily functions, including regulating metabolism and controlling blood sugar levels. However, chronic stress can lead to prolonged cortisol release, which may result in various health issues, such as anxiety, depression, and immune system suppression. After a brain injury, the HPA axis can become dysregulated, leading to imbalances in cortisol levels. This imbalance can exacerbate feelings of stress and overwhelm, making it even more crucial to find healthy ways to manage stress.

Stress Dosage

You may be asking, what is the **right dosage of stress for me?** Well, I hate to be that guy, but it is impossible to guess without me knowing what your individual life factors are. Stress is not only physical but also mental, emotional, social, and spiritual. This is why you can do tests on identical twins with very similar life experiences, and they will react completely differently to any given stressor. **If we see the stressor as something positive that is helping us grow vs something that is horrible for us, we will have a completely different reaction to it.**

After a brain injury, your nervous system is thrown off balance and homeostasis, which makes even small stressors feel overwhelming. This is where hormesis comes in. By gradually building up stress tolerance, we strengthen our resilience and work our way back to a healthy baseline.

It's all about gradually raising our stress threshold and increasing our resilience.

Just like we lift weights, we want to do so in a manner of progressive overload, the same goes for stress. We want to gradually increase the amount we can take.

Take Action Today

Take a cold shower. Depending on how stressful your life is right now, I want you to push a little past your current limits. If you already are used to cold showers, maybe make it a little colder by doing an ice bath or try to increase the amount of time that you stay in by 30 seconds.

If it's your first time, maybe simply getting in for 30 seconds will do it for you. Remember, it's all about finding that balance and harnessing the power of the right amount of stress.

Your VIP Invitation Is Here! Early access, huge savings, and 15 free Mind Gym Memory-boosting exercises are just a scan away or go to www.dr-bro.com/vipbrainrescue

CHAPTER NINE: THE SIXTH PILLAR: N IS FOR N.E.X.U.S

You have now entered the **NEXUS** point of your journey. The word "NEXUS" means **connection**. It's the point where different things meet and converge, creating a powerful system.

My studies at the International Quantum University of Integrative Medicine with professionals like Dr. Bruce Lipton, Gregg Braden, Dr. Joe Dispenza, Dr. Patrick Porter and Nassim Harramein have opened my mind to the fact that everything is interconnected. Learning these ideas will help you understand the bigger picture of your recovery. I admit some of them may seem a bit complex at first, but if an ex-college drop out can learn them, then I promise so can you...

THE FIRST STEP IS N FOR NONLOCALITY:

> "There's A Natural Mystic Flowing Through The Air"
>
> — BOB MARLEY

You ever feel like what you're doing doesn't matter? Like the world's just too big, and you're too small to make any kind of difference? Let me hit you with the truth right now: Everything you do matters. It matters big time, and not just to the people around you but to the entire universe. This is called non-locality. The Universe works in "non-local" ways because everything is interconnected. If you have ever heard of a black hole, it is a vortex to which space and time cannot even escape. This is what happens when you get deep into the present moment or into a flow state. There is no time, there is no space. There only is...

Einstein believed that the past, present, and future are interconnected. He said; "The distinction between past, present and future is only a stubbornly persistent illusion".

But here's the catch: just because you do not see, hear, smell, feel, sense or touch something, does not mean that it doesn't exist. In fact, what we perceive is only a small percentage of reality.

How Non-Locality Shows Up in Everyday Life

Think about how quickly people judge others today, especially on social media. You see one post, one photo, or one comment, and suddenly you think you know someone. But what you're seeing is just the surface, a small slice of a much larger picture. The same goes for how we perceive ourselves and the impact we have on the world. Non-locality teaches us to pause, to see beyond the obvious, and to recognize the deeper, unseen connections at play. Every action, no matter how small, reverberates across this web of connection. When you focus on the positive, you're not just changing your own energy—you're influencing the entire system.

Why This Matters to You

Understanding non-locality isn't just a cool theory; it's a mindset for transformation. It means that even on your toughest days, when symptoms feel overwhelming or progress feels slow, what you do still matters. Each intentional breath, each kind thought, each step forward creates ripples of healing not just in you but in the world around you. So before you judge yourself or someone else based on what you see in a single moment, remember this: you're part of something bigger. And every choice you make has the power to change it.

THE SECOND STEP IS E FOR ENTANGLEMENT:

> *"To Tap The Force Of The Universe Itself, We Must See Ourselves As Part Of The World Rather Than Separate From It"*
>
> — GREGG BRADEN

Have you ever wondered why a mother can sense when something is wrong with her child? **How she *just knows*, even if they're halfway across the world?** There's no phone call, no text, yet she feels it deep in her gut. Why? Because even though they're separated in space and time, they are still connected in a way most people can't explain. It's not magic, it's called quantum entanglement, my friends. You see, when two particles become entangled, it doesn't matter if they're inches apart or light-years away—what happens to one instantly affects the other. Instantly! Change the state of one particle, and the other responds immediately. There's no lag time, no waiting around. It even happens faster than the speed of light. That's the power of entanglement, and you better believe it applies to people too. But don't just take my word for it—this isn't some fairy tale idea.

I am going to refer to Nicolas Gisin's study once again that pushed this from a theory into hard science. His team proved this connection was real by separating entangled particles with a laser, sending them 10 kilometers apart through fiber optic cables. They showed the particles still responded to each other faster than light could travel. Imagine that for a second—no matter the distance, they were still linked, still reacting to each other in real-time! Even though conventional thinking states that particles are separate and have no communication with one another, they act as if there still connected.

This experiment wasn't done once, it's been tested and retested.

Now here's where it gets even more real. This isn't just some fancy laboratory experiment either. This is life. This is you, me, and everyone you've ever been connected to. This is karma, this is the universe's cosmic balancing act. Every action you take, every word you speak, creates an energy, a ripple. And like entanglement, that energy doesn't fade just because it's out of sight. It's coming back to you, whether it's tomorrow, next week, or in a decade—it's on its way.

So if you're out there throwing negativity into the world—spreading hate, being mean, acting out of selfishness—don't think for a second you're immune from what's coming.

That's because every action has an equal and opposite reaction! There's no getting around that!

Once something is joined, it is always connected, whether it remains physically linked or not.

So don't take this lightly. The universe is watching, reacting, and responding to every move you make. You are not just a drop in the ocean. You are the ocean in a drop. Every ripple you send out affects the whole. The law of entanglement, karma, energy—call it what you want—it's all the same. What you give, you get back. Make sure you're giving something worth receiving.

THE THIRD STEP IS X FOR X-RAY:

> *The Beauty Of The Electromagnetic Spectrum Is That It Contains All Forms Of Light. What We Can See Is Just A Tiny Sliver Of It."*
>
> — NEIL DEGRASSE TYSON

You are stuck in the matrix. But not in the same way that you think.

As mentioned before, we only perceive a small percentage of reality, and I am going to prove that to you. Let's consider an X-ray machine, for example. Look at a picture of the electromagnetic spectrum below. The X-ray machine emits radiation at wavelengths of about 0.01 to 10 nanometers. This means that the X-ray's energy is much higher than visible light, which is why we cannot see it with the naked eye.

Now, look at the colors we can see, part of the visible light spectrum:

- Red has a wavelength of approximately 620 to 750 nanometers.
- Orange is around 590 to 620 nanometers.
- Yellow is between 570 to 590 nanometers.
- Green is around 495 to 570 nanometers.
- Blue ranges from 450 to 495 nanometers.
- Violet (Purple) is approximately 380 to 450 nanometers.

Similarly, the same principle applies to sound. Humans can hear sound frequencies between 20 Hz and 20,000 Hz (20 kHz), but most sounds are beyond our hearing range…

The same is true for all our senses like smell and touch.

Different animals can perceive different things. Have you ever heard of a dog whistle?

It's a small whistle that humans can't hear, but dogs can! That's because the sound it makes is at a frequency higher than what our ears can pick up. While we hear nothing, dogs can hear it loud and clear.

Their sense of smell is estimated to be between 10,000 to 100,000 times more acute than ours.

This shows us that we are only capable of perceiving a small fraction of the full electromagnetic spectrum, while many other frequencies, like X-rays and ultraviolet light, exist beyond what we can perceive. The reality we perceive is just a tiny slice of the full spectrum!

So your ability to tune into different energies and vibrations is always changing. When you change what you focus on and your daily habits, this changes, like the reticular activating system I was telling you about before!

This is directly related to how our **memories** work. The more in touch you are with the energy and frequency of your vibration, the easier you can recall that memory.

You're remembering only a fraction of what's possible for your mind!

This is how you **Rescue Your Brain!** Your brain is a **frequency-detecting machine!** The better it works the more you can tune into!

Change your energy, change your life!

THE FOURTH STEP IS U FOR UNKNOWN:

> *"The Best Way To Predict The Future Is To Create It"*
>
> — DR. JOE DISPENZA

Listen up, because I'm about to drop some truth on you that most people are too scared to face. Do you want your **memory** back? You want to stop feeling lost in your own head, wondering if you'll ever be the same? Then you better be ready to do what most people won't. Get used to the uncertainty and OWN it.

Ever heard of the Uncertainty Principle? It came from a study by **Werner Heisenberg** in **1927**, and its **pretty crazy**. Heisenberg was a physicist who was exploring the behavior of tin particles, like electrons. He wanted to measure both were they were (position) and how fast they were moving (momentum). He found something straight up mind blowing. That you can't know where a particle is and how fast it's moving at the same time. The more precisely you try to measure one, the less accurately you can measure the other. It's a big part of quantum mechanics, but we're not here to talk science, we're here to talk your memory.

Life and recovery are like that, too. Right now, you're trying to figure out where your memory is, trying to grab it and fix it. But here's the truth. You can't force it back into place. Your brain, just like those tiny particles in Heisenberg's principle, won't respond to being forced into a box. You try to push it too hard, and suddenly everything feels uncertain or like it's slipping away.

But guess what? That's okay. Because the real power comes in accepting that uncertainty. You're not going to get all the answers right away, and that's part of the process. You're not here to be perfect every second of the day. You're here to move forward, inch by inch, and that's where the real strength comes from.

Perfection doesn't exist. In fact, the more you try to do things perfectly, the more you are going to struggle. It's important to accept our imperfections and learn to make mistakes in life because mistakes are the best learning lessons that life gives us. Take, for example, when you first learned to ride a bicycle. You fell again and again. It was horrifying. But you eventually got to that beautiful moment in time when everything came together, and you were riding! That's the essence of life and learning! Mistakes are really just small samples of life.

Don't just read it! Apply it!

1. **Forget perfection.** You're not going to nail every detail right now. Stop expecting it. Every time you try to grab onto something perfectly, you're only tightening the noose around your own progress. Accept the imperfections of life.
2. **Face the uncertainty** head-on. You don't know when everything will come back. And you know what? Good. That's where the real warriors rise. You don't need everything to be certain to dominate your life. You need to show up, even when the path is unclear, and keep hammering away.
3. **Take action every damn day.** Memory comes back to those who WORK for it. Do the exercises, write things down, practice meditation, and push your limits. You're going to feel stuck sometimes but do it anyway. Get up and take a swing, no matter how off-target you feel. No excuses.

Most Worriers love to whine about uncertainty. You're not one of them. You're a Warrior who thrives in it. The more you push forward without needing everything to be perfect, the more unstoppable you become. It's not about getting your memory back in one big moment. It's about showing up and fighting for it each and every day. You don't need it all to be clear—you just need to MOVE. So, stop overthinking and make it happen. Embrace the chaos and keep driving forward. Get after it.

THE FIFTH STEP IS S FOR SUPERPOSITION

> *"Life Is Not A Window; It's A Mirror!"*
>
> — WES WATSON

In the quantum world, particles like electrons or atoms exist in a state of **superposition**, meaning they can be in multiple places at the same time. This is the ultimate reflection of how our lives unfold. We are not confined to one path or one possibility. At any given moment, we are simultaneously existing in different states—fear, hope, success, and doubt.

In other words, reality performs in both a particle and a wave.

The Famous Double Slit Experiment

Picture this: you have a light source that shoots tiny particles, like electrons, toward a barrier with two narrow slits in it. You'd expect those particles to go through one slit or the other, right? But when they hit the screen behind the barrier, you don't see just two lines. Instead, you see a strange pattern of stripes. So, what's happening here? The particles are acting like waves. They're going through both slits at the same time and mixing together, just like waves in water creating ripples. It's wild! Now, here's the jaw-dropper: if you set up a detector to find out which slit the particles actually went through, everything changes. The moment you try to check, the cool wave pattern disappears, and you only see two lines on the screen again. It's like the particles are saying, "You're watching? Okay, I'll act like a regular particle!"

This experiment shows us something mind-blowing: **observation changes reality**. Before you look, the particles can be in many different states. But the instant you measure them, they choose one. It's a powerful reminder that what you focus on can shape your world in ways you might not even know!

The double-slit experiment has been conducted by various researchers over the years, consistently confirming wave-particle duality:

1. **Thomas Young (1801):** First demonstrated that light can create an interference pattern when passing through two slits.
2. **Claus Jönsson (1961):** Showed that electrons also produce interference patterns, indicating they behave as both particles and waves.
3. **Modern Variations:** Recent experiments have tested the phenomenon with atoms and molecules, reinforcing that wave-like behavior also extends to larger particles.

If you want a short, but great understanding of this concept, I suggest you search YouTube for the video "Dr. Quantum Double Slit".

Syntropy And Entropy

Gazing at the Stars: Understanding Our Universe Through Syntropy and Entropy

When you look up at the night sky, what do you see? Countless stars twinkling against the vast darkness of the universe. Each star represents a story of creation, destruction, and everything in between. This cosmic dance relates to two main ideas. Things are always coming together through **syntropy,** and things are always falling apart through **entropy**.

Entropy: Things Fall Apart

In the universe, **entropy** is about how things move from order to disorder. For instance, stars are born, live for millions or even billions of years, and eventually die, often in spectacular explosions called supernovas. After these explosions, the elements created can mix into the universe, leading to new stars and planets. This cycle shows us that while entropy increases over time, leading to more chaos, it also creates the conditions for new beginnings. It's like a reminder that even in the messiness of life, new opportunities can emerge. Just as stars evolve, our minds can experience chaos after a brain injury but can also find pathways to healing and renewal.

Syntropy: Things Come Together

Now, think about **syntropy**, which is the movement toward organization and connection. When you look at a constellation, for example, you're seeing a group of stars that, from our perspective on Earth, forms a pattern. These patterns symbolize the connections we can make in our own lives. In the universe, syntropy encourages collaboration and balance. For example, gravity pulls stars together, forming galaxies, while the energy from stars fuels the growth of planets. This interplay between chaos and order shows that even when things seem overwhelming, there's a natural push toward healing and structure.

The universal laws of **syntropy** and **entropy** are closely connected to memory recovery after a brain injury. Just as the universe experiences cycles of chaos and order, our minds also navigate through moments of confusion and clarity. After an injury, it may feel like memories are scattered and disorganized—reflecting entropy. However, by embracing syntropy, people can create new connections and pathways in their brains, much like how stars form constellations. Through practices like mindfulness, creativity, and community support, you can foster order from chaos, facilitating a journey toward healing and a more resilient memory.

> **Your VIP Benefits Are Waiting!** Unlock huge discounts, exclusive offers, and free tools to reclaim your memory. Go to www.dr-bro.com/vipbrainrescue or scan below.

CHAPTER TEN: THE SEVENTH PILLAR: D IS FOR D.E.D.I.C.A.T.E

This is the last stage but definitely not the least important part of the program. Now that you have all the tools that work, it is time to dedicate to using them for the rest of your life.

I can show you the door, but it's up to you to walk through it.

THE FIRST STEP IS D FOR DISCIPLINE:

> *"Discipline is Freedom"*
>
> — JOCKO WILLINK

When it comes down to it, are you willing to show up every day, no matter how you feel, and put in the work? If you're serious about recovery, you must teach your brain that you are serious. **Discipline is a daily spiritual practice that sharpens the sword of your mind and memory.**

Lao Tzu said it best. "He who conquers others is strong; he who conquers himself is mighty."

Or as the modern-day poet ICE CUBE says it, "**You betta check yourself before you wreck yo-self!**" Jokes aside, your true power comes from inside. At a molecular level: recovery is war, and discipline is your weapon. I'm not sugarcoating this, what you're facing isn't just tough, it's brutal. But your brain is capable of more than you can imagine, and if you're willing to just push past your comfort zone, you'll find out just how adaptable you really are. This is going to require a kind of discipline that's not just about showing up when it's easy but showing up when every cell in your body is telling you to quit.

Let's talk straight science. When you commit to disciplined action, whether it's exercise, meditation, cognitive training, or just sticking to a routine, you're engaging the brain's neuroplastic mechanisms. **Every time you take action, no matter how small, you're triggering a cascade of neurochemical events that reinforce and strengthen synaptic connections. This is known as** *synaptic plasticity,* **and it's how neurons communicate more efficiently over time.** But it only works if you're consistent. The brain isn't going to waste energy rewiring itself for half-measures and occasional efforts. It demands relentless input to adapt, or else it will default to its old, damaged pathways. Bear with me, as I get a little geeky again. Synaptic plasticity is the basis of learning and memory and the first step in experience-dependent plasticity, improving the strength of connections. The second step involves the sprouting of new synapses, expressed in the nature of the dendritic spine.

Look, I realize that a lot of this may seem a bit tedious, redundant, and repetitive. This is because it needs to be said over and over again so that it will imprint upon your subconscious mind! These words will help create those pathways for your brain to implement what you have been learning, you need to understand the stakes here, we're talking about rewiring your brain down to the level of *gene expression.* Yes, you heard that right. The daily choices send signals to your cells that influence which genes get turned on or off. When you stay disciplined and train your brain to function under stress, you're actually changing the expression of genes that regulate stress resilience, inflammation, and even neurogenesis, the growth of new neurons. You're not just fighting your symptoms; you're reshaping the very biology of your recovery.

Cortisol, the stress hormone, gets a bad rap. In controlled amounts, but in the right amounts, it actually is what signals your brain to act and get moving. **I spoke about** *hormesis effect,* **where exposure to stress in manageable doses builds resilience.**

But let me be brutally honest: this isn't about half-hearted attempts of "maybe tomorrow." It's about showing up, whether your emotions feel ready or not. The brain has something called the default mode network, it's where your mind wanders, where self-doubt and negativity creep in. Left unchecked this becomes the breeding group for bad behaviors.

But when you choose discipline, when you engage in focused tasks, you're rewiring the default mode network. You're not giving your brain the luxury to wallow in what's not working; you're forcing it to adapt to what you do.

Discipline isn't punishment. It's LIBERATION! The more you lean into this, especially on the days when you feel broken, tired, or unsure, those are the moments that matter most. This is how you grab recovery by the horns and take the reins. This is how you move through the fog and break through it with trust and purpose. You have what it takes inside, Warrior!

ACTION STEP:

DEDICATE YOURSELF TO BECOMING A MORE DISCIPLINED PERSON IN YOUR LONG-TERM RECOVERY.

THE SECOND STEP IS E FOR: EDUCATE

> *Education Is The Most Powerful Weapon Which You Can Use To Change The World."*
>
> — NELSON MANDELA

It's time to **DEDICATE** to **EDUCATE** yourself and identify **as a** lifelong learner. The word educate is derived from the Latin **"educo,"** meaning to educe, to draw out, to **develop from within. In other words, you must first have the internal desire to educate yourself, and then act upon that.** This "missing link" of today's educational system is how they fail to teach students how to organize and use knowledge after they acquire it. **I'll tell you straight up, one of the biggest turning points in my own recovery was when I stopped acting like I had all the answers and started chasing knowledge like my life depended on it—because it did!** I remember hearing Tom Bilyeu from Impact Theory screaming at the top of his lungs, **"Be the learner!"**, over and over, **"I am the learner!"** I started repeating it myself.

This autosuggestion sunk deep into my subconscious mind. That wasn't just some feel-good mantra. It was a demand to never stop growing, to never stop pushing my mind.

And you know what? It worked! I don't even think about it now because I know that I am a lifelong learner, and **MAN has it paid off.** I used to think I was stupid, just a college dropout who would never amount to anything. **Now I am a learner and genius**! Once again, for the 100th time, all behavior is identity-based. You can do the same. Repeat these words or other affirmations as many times as necessary. It's all about mindset my friend. Make learning a lifestyle, stay curious, and watch how your **memory** expands.

Now, think about this: every piece of information you consume is a building block for your future. It's not just about **memory**; it's about empowerment. The more you learn, the more tools you have to face life's challenges. You become better equipped to adapt and overcome obstacles. You'll start to see the world differently, understanding the deeper connections between things, which only enhances your cognitive abilities.

You have the power to redefine yourself through knowledge. With every book you read, every lesson you learn, you're not just filling your brain—you're laying the foundation for a future that's brighter and more fulfilling than you ever thought possible.

Get obsessed with it. **Stay curious, stay hungry,** and you'll be unstoppable. That's how you make sure your memory, your mind, and your life don't just survive, but thrive.

Now go put in the work. **DEDICATE** to **EDUCATE** yourself every day.

Make this part of your mission and watch how your entire world changes for the better!

Action Step: DEDICATE yourself to learning 5 minutes minimum of daily learning, whether that is reading, listening to a podcast, or a YouTube video. Whatever is your preferred learning style. If you learn every day for 5 minutes, that is over 30 hours of learning in a year! That adds up! Imagine how much sharper your memory and skills will be. Because learning is neuroplasticity in action!

THE THIRD STEP IS D FOR DECIDE:

> *"Successful People Make Decisions Quickly And Change Them Very Slowly. Unsuccessful People Make Decisions Very Slowly, And Change Them Often And Quickly"*
>
> — NAPOLEON HILL

This next step to your long-term recovery is to firmly **DECIDE** to **DEDICATE** yourself to a long-term recovery. Sounds simple enough, right? But let me tell you, this is where most people get stuck. People have the horrible habit of being indecisive, thinking that that will help them make better choices if they just wait, analyze, and overthink. Wrong! **Second-guessing every move leads to a state of analysis paralysis.** You freeze up, and inaction destroys progress

In life, you're going to make mistakes. There's no escaping that. But here's the thing: you can get into the habit of making decisions quickly and with conviction to build momentum. And guess what? Momentum is the real key to success, not perfection.

The Power of Micro Decisions

Each day is made up of thousands of **micro-decisions** that either move you closer to or further from your recovery goals. **Each micro decision on its own makes no tangible difference in your life, but long term all of them collectively make a gigantic difference in the quality of your life.** Most people think short term and choose whatever is easiest and least painful in the moment. But **99% of the time, what feels easy and comfortable in the short term, is bad for you in the long term.** On the flip side, what is hard and uncomfortable in the short term, is good in the long run for you. The good news is you are 100% in control of making better decisions when you train yourself just do it.

Let's take diet and exercise for example. Every meal you eat, every choice to be active, and even how much you decide to eat might seem insignificant on their own, but together, these small choices create a powerful momentum. Choosing wholesome, nutrient-dense foods in satisfying but reasonable portions can support your energy and mental clarity, while avoiding the habit of overeating, helps keep you feeling lighter and more focused.

If you skip one workout or choose an unhealthy meal now and then, it might feel like no big deal. However, if this becomes a pattern, those choices can lead to a lack of progress or even setbacks in your recovery. On the other hand, consistently making a choice to nourish your body with balanced portions and prioritize movement, even on days when you don't feel like it, builds resilience and supports brain health over time.

The Brain Science of Decisions

Decisiveness is crucial for improving **memory**. Every time you make a decision you are training your brain. Every decision you make fires up new neural connections, strengthening your brain's capacity for memory and learning. What happens when you constantly second-guess yourself? Your brain stays stuck in disempowering patterns. You're not giving it a chance to grow and learn. "**Mistakes**" are the brain's way of learning. Our amazing cerebellum plays the role as our brain's error detection and correction mechanism. Think of the day that you learned to ride the bike once again? You fell and fell until your brain was like wow! The cerebellum says "oh well, we messed up a few things but, now we got this!" The same is true as when a baby eagle is learning to fly. If it doesn't learn to fly it will die! It has to have the courage to fail a few times until one day it soars!

The same is true for you!

Train yourself to be more decisive and trusting, regardless even if you "**fail**" Every choice you make, no matter how small, is an opportunity to create the person that you want to become. By making decisions quickly and confidently, you're forcing your brain to adapt, to learn from consequences, and ultimately to get stronger. And let me tell you something else. **"Mistakes" are the best teachers.** You're going to make wrong calls along the way. That's a given. But the faster you make those mistakes, the faster you can grow and learn. Mistakes aren't failures; they're stepping-stones It took **Thomas Edison** countless hours of trials with the lightbulb before he succeeded. He is quoted as saying. "**I have not failed. I've just found 10,000 ways that won't work.**" Accept that fact and apply it to your brain health recovery process.

I'm not saying to throw logic out the window completely. **Balance is key.** There are times when you need to slow down, assess, and weigh your options. But don't let that become your default.. The worst thing you can do is sit around, paralyzed by indecision, afraid of making the wrong choice. Inaction will keep you exactly where you are. In life, you are going to make "bad decisions. You will make **"mistakes"**. There is no way of getting out of that. But get in the habit of making them quickly and with a firm belief.

I get it. **Decision fatigue is real, and it's brutal.** The more decisions you leave lingering in your mind, the more energy you waste. Start making swift decisions and watch how much mental energy you free up. That's energy you can then use to push your recovery forward, to focus on strengthening your brain and sharpening your memory.

ACTION STEP: Start small. Start by making one fast decision every day. Maybe it's about your recovery routine, maybe it's about a habit you want to drop or a new strategy you want to try. Whatever it is, decide quickly and stick with it. See what happens when you commit.

Your long-term recovery is waiting for you. But it all starts with deciding to go all-in! Decide to be great. Decide to become unstoppable. Decide that you are worthy. Decide that you are going to win. Decide that you are going to stop making excuses. Decide that you are going to create an awesome life! No more hesitating, no more overthinking. Just bold, confident action. and that's how you win this fight. Trust in yourself; you've got this, Warrior! Now get out there and **DEDICATE** yourself to become a better decision-maker, and let your recovery take off like never before.

THE FOURTH STEP IS I FOR INTEGRATE:

> *"The Ability Of The Brain To Integrate information Is The Foundation Of Learning and Adaptation."*
>
> — DR. SIMON SCHULTZ

DEDICATE to INTEGRATE all that you learn,

Integration is our brain's process of converting short-term memories into long-term memories. When we learn new information or movements, we need to **integrate** them. We spoke about the importance of processing speed. The final step of the learning and converting memories into long-term storage is through integration. The steps look like this:

1. **Arrival:** New sensory info arrives to our brain.
2. **Processing:** Our brain processes what comes to us.
3. **Integration:** Our brain fully integrates things.
4. **Storage:** The learnings are stored away for later use.

Tools For Integration

With the one-on-one work and group coaching I do with my patients, I teach something called an **integration sandwich**. It starts with a quick 5-minute breathing session, followed by 30-35 minutes of brain exercises and learning, and end with 10-15 minutes of dynamic breathing.

Why do I do this? I do this because it drastically improves your ability to process and integrate what you have learned. This is important for several reasons. I mentioned in the past studies that prove how interconnected breathing and memory are. A remarkable study proves that when you breathe after following an exercise with breathing your brain sequences the same neural connections that you learned or preformed.

This is revolutionary! Let's take boxing for example. Let's say you worked really hard at the gym, correlating different combinations, hitting the jump rope for mobility, and you ending with the speed bag. When you end the session with a **deep dynamic breathing session** you are not only reducing stress levels, you are also forming new neural pathways, strengthening existing connections, as well as re-firing the sequences and patterns that you formed during the session!

It doesn't only apply to boxing. It can work with almost anything. Reading, studying, mind gym exercises… Whatever!

This may double the speed of processing and integrating new information.

THE FIFTH STEP IS C FOR CURIOSITY:

> *"We Keep Moving Forward, Opening New Doors, And Doing New Things, Because We're Curious, And Curiosity Keeps Leading Us Down New Paths."*
>
> — WALT DISNEY

Let's face it. **Our brain hates open loops**! Think of the last time you watched a movie or Netflix series, with all the drama and the ups and downs. The more suspenseful, the better! This is because **curiosity** is the deep itch you have to fill open loops. **Curiosity** significantly improves our ability to remember. One study proved this beyond any reasonable doubt, In the study, people rated how interested they were after receiving pop quiz questions about random pictures. It turned out that the more curious they were about the questions, the better they remembered. Brain scans showed that curiosity boosts dopamine activity in areas linked to reward and motivation (like the ventral striatum) and regions linked to memory (like the hippocampus).

Curiosity boosts dopamine levels a lot! Let me break it down in a way that hits home. **You see, dopamine is not your everyday neurochemical; it's a neuromodulator, meaning that it directly "modulates" (changes) behavior.** It creates a chemical cascade across multiple brain networks when ignited. When you're really curious about something, your brain acts like a sponge, soaking up not just what you're interested in but also other things around you. You're priming yourself to learn, grow, and elevate your game. Embrace that curiosity, and let it fuel your journey.

Once again, our brain hates open loops. It craves finality to any story. Curiosity helps fill those empty loops. We need to harness this and make it our mission to build our curiosity muscle. Stretch that curiosity muscle! Look for curiosity in everything----even in the mundane parts of life. Dive deep into your thoughts and emotions.

Curiosity and Confusion?

Embrace **CONFUSION**. Confusion is a good thing. You're probably thinking, wait a minute? How can that be? I hate being confused! Understand that there will be confusion before you can learn anything. And guess what! This is a great sign you are on the right track. **Confusion is simply new concepts fusing together.** When you look at how neuroplasticity and learning really works, you will understand that it can be a painful process when getting started. It will feel uncomfortable, you will feel frustration and doubt. This is an awesome part of your learning process because to truly learn, things need to be disassembled in your mind and put back together again so it makes sense!

Confusion just means it doesn't make sense to your current level of understanding. To change your results, you have to think in a different way! When you realize this, it's really simple. But for most people who can't or won't grasp this simple concept, they end up believing that it's their mind's way of telling them they can't or shouldn't do something.

Be **CURIOUS** with your **CONFUSION** and remember, confusion is actually a sign you are on the right track! Curiosity and confusion are signals of growth. Embrace curiosity to unlock new possibilities and welcome confusion as a sign you're on the right track. These aren't obstacles—they're steps toward deeper understanding. Stay curious, lean into the challenge, and keep moving forward. Your best discoveries lie ahead!

Boost Your Memory by Strengthening Your Curiosity Muscle

1. **Intent:** Set your Daily Intention to Be More Curious.
2. **Notice:** Pay attention to daily life situations with a sense of curiosity. Instead of reacting, just observe things with a sense of curiosity.
3. **Record:** Write down 3-5 things in your journal of things that were really interesting and provoked your curiosity.

THE SIXTH STEP IS A FOR ALIGNMENT:

> "Happiness Is When What You Think, What You Say, And What You Do Are In Harmony."
>
> — MAHATMA GANDHI

Alignment is everything. When you're in complete alignment with your highest self, you will create everything you desire in life. The universe, God.... Whatever your religious beliefs are, molds for those who truly listen to their calling. If your actions don't match your intentions, you're setting yourself up for disappointment and deep regret. If you don't get aligned, I guarantee you will **SABOTAGE** yourself. Whether that happens all in one night or slowly over time. It doesn't matter. **Please take my advice before you end up spending time in County Jail like I did!** I needed to understand the hard way to realize that I was literally not creating the person I saw in my head. I was not in alignment with the vision I had for myself.

Imagine trying to drive a car with misaligned wheels; you'll struggle to stay on the road, and that's exactly what happens when we lack alignment in our lives. When your thoughts, words, and actions are in sync, you create a powerful force that propels you forward. This congruence sharpens your memory and focus, allowing you to absorb and retain information like a sponge. If you are not aligned in your actions, you will create something very painful called cognitive dissonance. Cognitive dissonance occurs when your subconscious mind and conscious mind are in disagreement. Another way of seeing it is that your heart and brain disagree. This is a painful place to be in because it's like floating around in quicksand!

This is where alignment becomes your lifeline. When you are in alignment, you can unleash your full potential. Every decision you make should reinforce your goals and values, creating a clear path forward. No more wasted energy! Instead, you'll find clarity and focus, which will sharpen your memory and enhance your learning. We need to simplify our lives. Get back to the basics. Listen to the universe and take action in alignment with our future self.

How Aligned Are You?

To answer this question, first identify and find out what your deepest values are to see if you are aligned to them.

Action Step: 7 Steps to a Values Elicitation and Alignment Check

1. Determine a specific area of your life that you improve. Ex. Health, career, friendships etc.
2. Determine a specific goal, timebound, and actionable goal that you would like to achieve in this specific area. Example. I would like to acquire $5,000 by May 1st, by selling used cars.
3. Write down all of the values and desires for why you want to accomplish this goal. Example: I want more money because it will make me feel secure.
4. After you have identified, your values and desires for your goal, continuously ask yourself what are deepest reasons I want this value or desire? Ask questions, like what's important about (insert desire/reason?) Why do I want (insert desire/reason)?
5. Eventually, you will uncover a list of your highest and deepest values for your goal. Examples are love, joy, peace, wholeness, abundance. You will absolutely know when you have reached your highest values because when you ask the question, the value will repeat itself.
6. Check for alignment and congruence. Ask your subconscious mind. "Am I a loving person? Am I a joyful person? Etc.
7. If the answer is a "No or Maybe" and is not resounding or a definite yes, it a sign that you have some alignment work to do in this area. Repeat steps 1-7 of this process for best results.

THE SEVENTH STEP IS T FOR TASK-SWITCHING:

> *"Switching Between Tasks Takes A Toll On Your Brain, But The Ability To Do So Effectively Can Be Developed With Practice."*
>
> — ANDREW HUBERMAN

Imagine you're at a big party, and everyone is chatting, dancing, and having a blast. You are trying to have a deep conversation with your friend about the meaning of life while simultaneously keeping an eye on the nacho table, and notice that the delicious crispy nachos are almost completely gone.

How's that working out for you?

I think we all understand that focus is important for brain health, but so is the ability to switch between stimuli to stimuli.

This is called **cognitive flexibility...**

Ever watched a gymnast flip, twist, and turn mid-air? This is similar to the monumental stress your brain has to deal with to keep up with all the current distractions.

Every day seems like there's more pressure, distractions, and deadlines.

At the time of this current writing, we are just past the election season in the United States. The world seems to be moving to more divisiveness and distractions than ever before.

With all the fear, worry, doubt, and anxiety constantly creeping in, it's like having a mini-Olympics happening right inside your head.

But f*** that! **You can take your power back. The ball is in your court!**

You can use tough times to help be more flexible and resilient than ever before.

And that's where what I like to call "**brain yoga**" comes in. Just like stretching your muscles keeps your body limber, task switching, and cognitive flexibility keep your mind sharp. When you practice switching between different tasks with intention and focus, you're training your brain to handle anything that comes its way. You're building a kind of mental agility that allows you to move from one thing to the next without getting overwhelmed or losing your center.

Consistent practice at switching between tasks makes you stronger, sharper, and more capable of handling stress. **You're no longer a puppet to the distractions around you. Instead, you're fully in charge, moving through life with power and grace.** This is your superpower, your edge. You're not just keeping up with the distractions; you're rising above them.

Strengthening cognitive flexibility is like a mental workout. Think of it as "reps" for your brain: with each shift, you're training those mental muscles to handle more with less strain. Your brain can grow more adaptive with practice.

The Neuroscience of Task Switching

1. **Prefrontal Cortex (PFC):** This "executive center" helps with decision-making, problem-solving, and quickly shifting attention. The PFC allows us to focus on new tasks by blocking out irrelevant info and adapting our mental processing.

2. **Basal Ganglia:** This structure helps us identify patterns and manage habits. It sends signals to "switch gears" when we need to change tasks, helping us shift efficiently.

3. **Anterior Cingulate Cortex (ACC):** Acting as a feedback center, the ACC detects conflicts or errors and prompts the PFC to adjust focus as needed.

These areas together give us the mental agility to adapt, manage distractions, and stay focused amid disruptions.

Action Step: Use The Pomodoro Technique.

The **Pomodoro Technique** is a highly effective way to teach your brain to properly switch from one task to the next. It uses the principes of recency and primacy for learning the most effectively.

1. Choose 1 Task or Small Goal You Want To Accomplish.

2. Set a Timer for 25 minutes.

3. Take a Break.

- After each session, take a 5-minute break to reset.
- In that session, stretch. Do some squats or pushups. Then refocus yourself for the next 25-minute session.

THE EIGHTH STEP IS E FOR EMPOWERMENT:

> *"Empowerment Begins With The Choice To Believe In Yourself And The Courage To Take Action."*
>
> — TONY ROBBINS

Look, you've been through the storms and faced challenges that would crush most people. But here you are, still fighting, still pushing forward. **Empowerment** is the realization that your battle doesn't just build you; it makes you. Wake up, Warrior. It's time to own that power. The pain you've endured? None of that is in vain. You've felt weak, lost, beaten down, abandoned, maybe even like giving up. And guess what? That's exactly where your strength was born. That struggle? That wasn't there to break you; it was to help you dig deeper to show you exactly what you're made of. Too many people wait, hoping and waiting for the magic pill, a hack or the next "breakthrough." But empowerment? It means you're done waiting. You're done looking around for answers. **Because YOU are the ANSWER you have been searching for.** You're done being the victim in your own story. Empowerment is saying, "I'm my own savior and I am the creator of my life." The tough pill to swallow is that **if you don't learn how to empower yourself, the world will take advantage of you.** You are the one who can turn this around, no one else. That means embracing the struggles, the setbacks, the resistance and refusing to let it define you. You're done asking permission to heal, to move forward. You take that permission because it is your god-given right to. Refuse to let someone else take your power away.

Wake Your Inner GLADIATOR

Think about the moment in the movie **Gladiator** when **Maximus** gets in the arena to fight as a slave. **The once-great general has lost everything.** His family, his title, his pride, his freedom. **But how does he respond? He ultimately refuses to stay broken!** When he steps into the arena, he taps into something primal, something unbreakable. With every swing of his sword, every calculated move, he proves he's more than his circumstances. And then there's the moment when he stands before Emperor Commodus, the man who destroyed his life, and declares with unwavering defiance, "**My name is Maximus Decimus Meridius…and I will have my vengeance.**" He takes back his power. Not because it's easy but because it's beautiful.

Maximus reminds us of the universal truth. **No one can take away your internal power unless you let them win.** He didn't take pity upon himself. Instead, he used it as fuel in his belly for justice and redemption.

What makes this so special?

EVERY ADVERSITY, EVERY FAILURE, EVERY HEARTBREAK, CARRIES THE SEED OF AN EQUAL OR GREATER BENEFIT.

When you can view your failures objectively, you see what a gift they truly are.

You're able to seize them as an opportunity.

The seed of equal or greater benefit will be able to grow.

The more you allow it to grow, the stronger it will become.

Eventually, it will become larger than the failure from which it originally sprouted.

TAKE ACTION: THIS IS YOUR ARENA!

1-2-3 Process to DEDICATE to Long-Term EMPOWERMENT

1. **Commit to Growth**
   - Set a specific and measurable goal for yourself. Write it down and revisit it daily. Remind yourself why it matters and how achieving it will change your life.
2. **Create a Daily Empowerment Habit**
   - Incorporate one of more empowering activities into your daily routine. Whether it's journaling, meditation, or a morning mantra, consistency builds momentum.
3. **Track and Celebrate Progress**
   - Keep track of your wins, no matter how small. Celebrate each step forward and use it as fuel to keep going. Progress, not perfection, is the key to staying empowered.

Join the Movement! VIP members get exclusive early access to life-changing discounts and 15 free mind gym exercises. Scan the QR code or visit www.dr-bro.com/vipbrainrescue

CHAPTER ELEVEN: BRAIN INJURY WARRIORS. "STORIES OF HOPE!"

(How Ordinary People Completely Turned Their Life Around after Traumatic Brain Injuries and How You Can Too!)

Case Study #1 (Christina)

Christina, 31 (not her real name), works as a pharmacy assistant full-time. Many years before Christina came to see us, she was diagnosed with a calcification in her brain that was causing tonic-clonic seizures. Her whole life started unraveling and she really took a huge hit to her self-esteem. She discovered me online and found out about my history of seizures and had some questions to ask. It wasn't long before we started working together. My teachings about neuroplasticity and the power of the mind really got her attention dialed in. She consistently applied what I asked her to do within the R.E.B.O.U.N.D. method. She stopped watching excessive Netflix, changed her diet, started to exercise, meditate, breathe, and started taking targeted supplements to support her brain. Within a timeframe of 90 days, she reported feeling much better with 50% less fear and anxiety of her symptoms and diagnosis. These changes, along with strategies to improve Christina's sleep, caused her to say, "I feel so much more calm-minded". She went on to say, "The overthinking I used to do stopped a lot. Dr. Brody's very calm and collected. There's definitely a lot of understanding, a lot of sympathy, because of what he's been through. I'd say it's very positive and heartwarming. I'm definitely happy with our sessions, how far I've come, and the journey we have been taking". In the O.P.T.I.M.I.Z.E. portion of working together, we tripled Christina's reading speed from 204 words per minute to 615 words per minute. She went on to say about this… "It's been really good with remembering numbers! For some reason, when I would see a number only for a couple of seconds, I would still remember it. So, I think it's been really great for my memory!"

Case Study #2: Survivor to Thriver!

I'm Ryan Nurse, a traumatic brain injury survivor and thriver. Back in 2011, at the age of 18, I was attacked on the way home from a nightclub, which ultimately left me fighting for my life! I managed to make it back to my parent's house in the early hours after the attack and went straight to bed; however, later that Sunday morning, they failed to wake me up, and I was immediately rushed to the hospital. I needed an emergency brain operation as I suffered from a fractured skull and a blood clot due to a bleed on the brain. I was put into an induced coma on a life support machine, and the specialists told my parents it would be highly unlikely that I would make it through the night.

After three days in the coma, the specialists invited my parents to the hospital, and when they arrived, they were told to sit down and the surgeon said, "due to the severity of Ryan's injuries, and because there is absolutely zero brain activity when measured at the stem of his brain, we would highly suggest you consider switching off his life support machine." But in that moment, my dad instantly stood up and said, "NO FUCKING WAY! I own this machine, and I'll tell you when it gets turned off." He then went on to say, "I know Ryan more than any of you know him, and he takes his own time to do anything, so you need to give him that time." Because of what my dad did, they kept the machine on for a few more days, then decided it would be wise to reduce the sedation to bring me out of the coma. However, the morning the sedation was turned down, my lungs weren't functioning by themselves and I had to instantly be put back under sedation to stay in the coma. Again, the specialists told my parents that I was basically dead, and if I would somehow wake up from this, I would never walk or talk again and would be in a vegetative state for the rest of my life needing constant round the clock care and attention. But once again, my parents said no and that they needed to try again the next day. So they did, and thankfully for me my lungs did start to function, but now it was a waiting game to see what would happen.

After a week in a coma it was now time to see if I would come round or not, as doctors and specialists were constantly telling my loved ones that it would be highly unlikely I ever fully woke up. That second week it was said that I was making rapid progress, to the point that I was starting to hear and listen to what my friends and family were telling me. Then it got to the point where I would start making minimal movements of my toes and fingers after they told me to move them. This was fantastic news, and one day I actually opened my right eye after my nanny told me to. My parents were filled with hope, but the doctors immediately said it was all electrical impulses and I couldn't hear them. Just before I woke up fully, I was gifted an out of body/near-death experience where I witnessed myself in another dimension. This experience later led me to discovering my true life's purpose, and the real reason for why I'm here on this planet.

After all what the doctors and specialists predicted for my fate, I managed to wake up, learn to walk and talk again, and then leave hospital, all within less than four weeks. I never once took any medication or decided to carry on with any ongoing support both physically and mentally. They said I was a "walking miracle" as things like this don't happen. Of course, I suffered from extreme fatigue, and I had short-term memory loss for a while. However, this was nothing compared to what they had previously predicted. So, with all this being said, please don't let your diagnosis be your prognosis because no doctor could ever put a definite deadline on your dreaded day of demise. They can only give you information from their own knowledge and experience. But the thing is, we as humans are all unique individuals who heal and recover at our own pace. So when doctors say, you won't be able to do *this*, or you can't do *that* anymore after your brain injury, I would seriously take their advice with a pinch of salt, always listen to yourself, and do your own due diligence. Seek out guidance from others who have had the same injuries as you, and overcome the same challenges as you, then learn exactly how they did it. But whatever you do, don't let someone else decide, design, determine, or dictate your destiny.

I believe what helped me heal at a rapid rate, was that not once did I ever think or believe that I would be stuck the way I was forever. I never thought I'd be in hospital forever, I never thought I wouldn't be able to walk again, and I later went on to setting many goals and visions to focus on for the future. This was super important because what you focus on in life expands, if you think you can or think you can't you are right, and it's always progress that equals happiness. If I would have chosen to be a victim of my situation and stay stuck where I was, you would never be reading these words right now. So, realize that sometimes your most profound periods of pain can also turn out to be your greatest gifts of growth. Whatever has happened, has happened, and with the right support, who knows, just maybe, you can use your current challenge as your superpower in the near future. I'd really start to visualize your very best self within your own mind every day, because every single thing that has ever been created, has been created twice. That's once in the mind, and once in reality. See yourself living your best life when you *do* finally find the answers to overcome your current obstacles, and then make moves towards that life on a daily basis.

Doctors said I'd never be the same again, and when I think about it, they were right. Today I am stronger, smarter, and happier than I've even previously been. Through my pain I've found my passion and purpose. I've done and am still doing things they said I'd never be able to do. I'm positively impacting and inspiring lives all around the world through my words and actions, especially on my social media. I've published one book (Sort Your S-H-I-T Out!) and the second (Dying with Regrets) and many more are coming next. So please don't underestimate the power of your potential. Use my journey as hope and inspiration that *you* too have the power within you to comeback stronger than ever before!

Follow me on social media @Ryannurse_

Grab a copy of my books "SORT YOUR S-H-I-T OUT!" and "DYING WITH REGRETS"

Case Study #3 Kyle's Close Call

Kyle (not his real name) lived for the thrill of competition. A natural athlete, he quickly rose to the top of his sport, competing in international events and inspiring fans worldwide with his effortless skill and undeniable drive. He had his eyes set on a major competition and was only days away from achieving his biggest dream when a split-second miscalculation during a practice changed everything. What was supposed to be a routine maneuver went terribly wrong, and Kyle's fall left him with a severe traumatic brain injury, rendering him unconscious. His world, once defined by speed and power, was suddenly plunged into silence and uncertainty.

When he finally awoke from a coma, Kyle faced a terrifying new reality: he struggled with basic memory, had difficulty forming sentences, and couldn't recognize parts of himself he once knew so well. It was like being a stranger in his own mind; every simple task was now a Herculean challenge. He found himself grappling with emotions he'd never felt before frustration, despair, even a fear he couldn't shake that his life as he knew it was over. His athletic future was put on hold indefinitely, and doctors warned that he might never regain his former self, physically or mentally. Friends and family gathered around him, but the journey ahead was one he would largely have to face alone, in the depths of his own mind. For Kyle, the hardest part of recovery wasn't the physical challenges but the mental endurance it required. Progress was painfully slow, often discouraging. Some days, he could hardly remember what he'd done just hours earlier. Simple tasks exhausted him, and he felt trapped in a body and mind that no longer felt like his own. There were days he wondered if it was even worth it to keep pushing forward, haunted by the shadows of his past achievements.

But beneath the fear and frustration, a spark of his old competitive spirit remained. Kyle knew that quitting had never been an option in his sport, and he resolved that it wouldn't be an option in his recovery either. He dove into his rehabilitation with the same tenacity he had once reserved for competition, embracing neuroplasticity—the brain's remarkable ability to heal and rewire itself. He poured hours into cognitive and physical therapy, focusing on exercises to retrain his brain, regain his memory, and restore basic motor skills.

Kyle clung to every small victory: the day he could string together a few sentences, the first time he recognized the subtle contours of his face in the mirror, the moment he was able to hold a conversation without losing his train of thought. Each milestone, though tiny, fueled his drive to keep going. Months turned into years, and though progress was slow, he discovered new parts of himself that were even stronger and more resilient than he'd ever known. The journey became less about returning to who he was and more about embracing who he could become.

Eventually, Kyle's dedication and resilience allowed him to return to his sport—not as a competitor but as a mentor and coach. He found a renewed purpose in guiding young athletes through the challenges of high-level competition and, most importantly, educating them on the importance of brain health and safety. His message was simple but powerful: "Protect the mind; it's the greatest asset you have.

Today, Kyle is a fierce advocate for brain injury awareness and the power of neuroplasticity. He's shared his journey with audiences worldwide, inspiring others who face the same darkness he once did. His story has become a beacon of hope for those who feel lost in their recovery, a living testament to the resilience of the human spirit. He reminds people everywhere that while recovery may seem impossible, healing is always within reach.

Kyle's journey proves that no matter how daunting the road, hope and perseverance can make the impossible possible. From the darkest of days to the brightest of triumphs, he's shown that true strength isn't about avoiding hardship; it's about finding a way through it.

Case Study #5 Dayana. My Story of Hope

Now I understand the diamond phrase you have to go through. When you're in a moment of pain, remember that it's a moment of transformation; this pain is pushing you to grow, to change your shape. I now see all the pain the butterfly endured, each change, each transformation that led it to its fullest potential. It took it to the ecstasy of flight, with all the changes it endured engraved on its wings, making it even more beautiful. This is your moment of transformation, your moment to become who you are truly meant to be. I'm learning to accept my new version, my new 'avatar,' more magical, more unique. I'm still learning, growing, crying, but always moving forward. I don't know exactly where I'm going, but I'd rather feel excited than worried about where life is leading. My transformation began in 2020, from a car accident and a brain injury.

Love you all. You can find me at @dayanalopezfamilyconstellation

AFTERWORD

The Power of Being a Human Being

Fantastic job, Warrior! You made it to the end of the book. This is a big deal! **If I were there with you in person, I would give you a huge high five**, so let's pretend I'm doing it anyway. So, give me an imaginary high-five right now! Not by chance, not by a stroke of luck, but through commitment, and the power within you to rise above. This moment isn't just finishing another book, it's a testament to your resilience, grit, and your belief in the possibility of change.

I hope you understand now the fact that nothing in this world is more important than your brain health! Not even 100's of millions of dollars! Along the way, we've explored the incredible potential of the brain to heal, adapt and thrive when you choose to believe in your ability to recover. The tools you've learned here aren't temporary fixes, they're foundations for a lifetime. They are here to help you rebuild, to rewire, to reclaim the life you deserve.

Let's take a moment to revisit the **7 Step Process called the R.E.B.O.U.N.D. Method**—the blueprint to follow for a successful recovery. Use the actionable steps you can carry forward with trust and confidence.

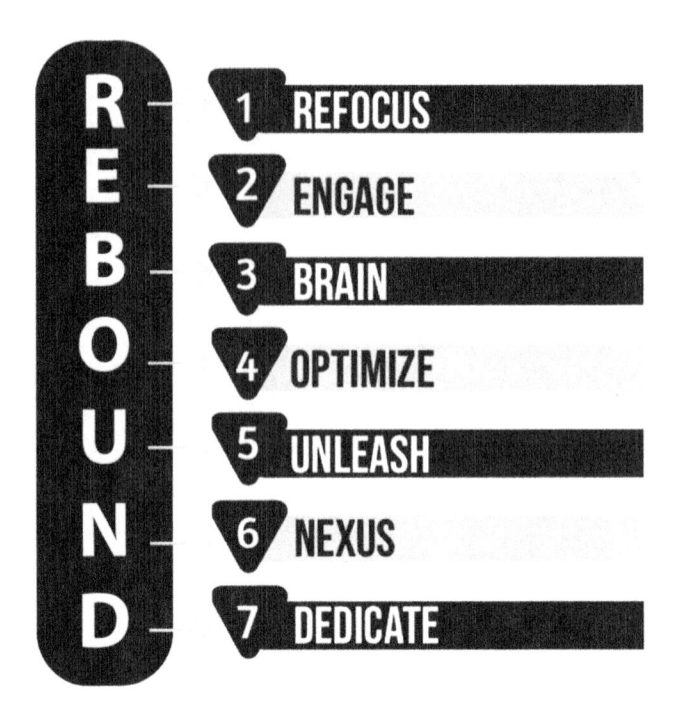

R — 1 REFOCUS
E — 2 ENGAGE
B — 3 BRAIN
O — 4 OPTIMIZE
U — 5 UNLEASH
N — 6 NEXUS
D — 7 DEDICATE

1. R.E.F.O.C.U.S.

Begin your recovery by building a strong foundation. **REFOCUS** your energy on the essentials—**rest, exercise, fuel, observation, consistency, understanding and supplementation.** These are the foundational steps that help stabilize you in the early stages of recovery, helping you regain mental strength and resilience. Without this groundwork, it's hard to build lasting progress in memory recovery.

2. E.N.G.A.G.E.

Dive deeper and start **ENGAGING** pathways that lead to long-term change.

Experience the power of activating both your brain and body in recovery. Harness **nitric oxide breathing** to supercharge your energy and healing potential. Cultivate **gratitude**, activate the **anterior**

cingulate cortex through doing hard things, **observe** yourself in the present moment. **Gamify** your recovery process to stay motivated and energized.

While making sure to **Emotionalize** helps engage the foundation for long-term and lasting changes in your brain health.

3. B.R.A.I.N.

Master the five principles of neuroplasticity: **breath, repetition, association, intensity, and novelty**. These principles are like tools in your recovery toolbox, allowing you to reshape your mind and create lasting, transformative changes.

4. O.P.T.I.M.I.Z.E.

Optimize your brain health to the next level by cultivating **optimism**, enhancing your **processing speed**, and refining **reaction timing**. Practice your ability of **inhibition**, using targeted **mind gym** exercises and improve balance through **inner ear** training. Create a space with **zero distractions** and align your progress by surfing your **emotions**. This step takes you beyond healing into a thriving state.

5. U.N.L.E.A.S.H.

Unleash your true potential by utilizing your **unconscious brain** and strengthening neural pathways. Activate your nervous system, detoxing your body through lymphatic flow, and incorporate that Energy-Enhancement System (EES) into your routine. Build focus through attention training and unlock faster learning through super learning techniques. Lean into hormesis, small, controlled challenges that push you to grow over time. Break through mental barriers and **unleash** your inner genius.

6. N.E.X.U.S.

Discover the **NEXUS.** of how you're interconnected to the world around you. By understanding principles from quantum physics, like energy fields and entanglement, you can learn to shape your reality and align your life with your highest intentions. Explore the power of **nonlocality** and how your brain interacts with the world beyond physical boundaries. Recognize the **entanglement**, the interplay between your thoughts, actions, and the energy around you. Remember the **x-ray** machine, the electromagnetic spectrum, and how everything is beyond what it seems. Embrace the **unknown**, where growth and discovery unfold. Step into a state of **superposition**, holding possibilities as you align your reality.

7. D.E.D.I.C.A.T.E.

Fully **DEDICATE** yourself to a long-term recovery. Begin to create the daily **discipline** and structure to reclaim your memory. Dedicate to **educate** yourself to become the identity of the learner. Have the patience and determination to **integrate** and process what you learn. Cultivate a deeper sense of **curiosity** throughout life's wild journey. **ALIGN** your thoughts and actions with the person you want to become. Become aware of the remarkable ability of how your brain **task switches,** but more importantly, learn how to **empower** yourself, because if you don't the world will gladly disempower you.

Commit to lifelong growth and empowerment. **Dedication** isn't just about recovery; it's about building a life full of purpose and possibility.

Congratulations on making it to the end of the book! Make sure to reread it to fire and wire new brain pathways because repetition is the mother of all learning!

I hope you can now fully grasp **how amazing your 100 billion dollar brain is!** Once again contact and combat sports athletes are starting to wake up to the fact that not even all the money in the world is more impor-tant than what's sitting in between their skull! This journey doesn't end with these pages. Recovery isn't a single destination; it's a daily journey to strengthen your mind, body, and spirit. Imagine the version of yourself that's free from limitations, living fully, and connected to their deepest potential. That version of you exists, and it's within reach. Keep going, not just for where you are now, but for the person you're becoming. Remember, you are more than just a body, more than just a mind. You're a force, a powerful, boundless energy that exists beyond the physical. Every day you have the power to choose. With each new choice, you create new neural pathways, reshaping your mind and reclaiming your freedom. This is the power of neuroplasticity—the power to literally rewire your brain, to make each thought, each action, and each belief work for you. You are the architect of your life, and you hold the keys to your own transforma-tion. The practices you've learned here—visualization, movement, meditation—are not just routines. Each one activates a different part of your brain. Visualization lights up the occipital lobe, action engages the prefrontal cortex and motor cortex, and positive self-talk strengthens your language centers. These aren't random exercises. They're designed to stimulate, awaken, and fortify the incredible capacities within you. Together, they bring you closer to the freedom and strength you're reclaiming.

Here's the choice: keep moving forward. **DEDICATE** fully, with no turning back. This is your moment. You've been given the tools, the knowledge, and the power. Now it's time to apply it. Step by step, thought by thought, action by action, make the choice to rise. Build the life you want. You're no longer at the mercy of your past or your limitations. This is your journey, and it's time to step into the version of yourself that's waiting on the other side.

BONUS CHAPTER

Mastering Memory Mechanics

Congratulations to all the Seekers out there who want to dive deeper. You've made it to the bonus chapter! If you're here, it's because you are as fascinated by the depths of the mind as I am.

First, there's **declarative memories,** our "knowledge bank." It holds the following:

- **Episodic memory**: personal memories, like vivid snapshots of moments in your life.
- **Semantic memory**: factual knowledge, like knowing that Paris is the capital of France.
- **Prospective memory**: Future memories, like remembering things we to do things in the future, like going to an appointment.

But memory isn't just about facts and events!

There are also **non-declarative memories**, a "hidden" kind of memory that includes:

- **Procedural memory**: skills you've practiced, like riding a bike or typing.
- **Emotional memory**: how we react based on past feelings and experiences.
- **Innate memory**: reflexes and automatic responses.

Each type of memory plays a part in how we learn, react, and recover.

In this chapter, we'll unpack each type, looking at how they function, where they're stored, and most importantly, how we can strengthen and work with them during brain recovery. You'll learn why these memories are foundational to who we are and how, with the right approach, we can reinforce, rebuild, and even relearn aspects of memory.

Ready to explore the next layer? Let's dive in!

Declarative Memory: The Brain's Active Archive

Declarative memory, also known as "explicit memory," is what we use when we actively try to remember. It includes two main types:

Episodic Memory: This is like a personal photo album. It helps us recall details about experiences we've had—like our first day of school, a special vacation, or a big accomplishment. Episodic memory is closely tied to emotions and senses, which is why certain smells or sounds can bring back memories. For people recovering from brain injuries, strengthening episodic memory can help them reconnect with important moments in their lives.

Research Insight: The prefrontal cortex plays a huge role in the retrieval of episodic memories; research studies have found greater Position Emission Tomography (PET) measurements of regional cerebral blood flow in the prefrontal cortex as the subjects were engaged in memory retrieval. [43]

Semantic Memory: Think of semantic memory as your personal encyclopedia. It's where you store general knowledge, facts, and meanings. Unlike episodic memory, it isn't linked to personal experiences. Instead, it holds objective information like vocabulary, historical dates, math formulas, or famous places For people recovering from brain injuries, semantic memory can be disrupted, making it hard to recall basic facts or recognize words. Simple exercises, like memory games or learning new subjects, can help strengthen this "encyclopedia" of knowledge.

Research Insight: Semantic memory relies heavily on brain regions, including the left temporal lobe, which plays a major role in processing and storing factual information. Studies using functional Magnetic Resonance Imaging (fMRI) have shown that areas in the left hemisphere, especially the left anterior temporal cortex, are more active during tasks that require recalling general knowledge. For example, a study by Binder et al. (2009) found that when subjects were engaged in semantic memory tasks, there was increased blood flow to these regions, indicating their role in fact-based knowledge retrieval. [44]

Prospective Memory: This is the memory that allows us to remember to do things in the future, such as attending a meeting or taking medication. Prospective memory is often crucial for daily life, especially in recovery, as it helps individuals keep track of tasks that support healing and routine. It involves planning and goal setting, engaging the prefrontal cortex, which helps with the mental organization of future tasks. For those with brain injuries, prospective memory can be disrupted, making reminders and structured routines helpful tools.

Research Insight: Studies suggest that the prefrontal cortex and hippocampus are key in prospective memory, particularly for goal setting and planning future tasks. An fMRI study by McDaniel and Einstein (2000) found increased activation in these areas during tasks involving prospective memory, underscoring their role in time-based intentions. [45]

Why Declarative Memory Matters in Recovery: Declarative memory, especially episodic memory, is often impacted by brain injuries. Recovery involves not only re-learning and reinforcing these memories but also stimulating these pathways to encourage neuroplasticity—the brain's ability to reorganize and form new connections. Working with declarative memory can help rebuild the mental "files" that store both personal and factual information.

Non-Declarative Memory: The Brain's Invisible Skills

Non-declarative memory, also called "implicit memory," is the background system that powers our automatic skills and instincts. We rely on it without realizing, and it often stays strong even when other memory types are affected by injury. Here's how non-declarative memory breaks down:

1. Procedural Memory: This is our muscle memory—the skills we've practiced so much that they become automatic, like typing, riding a bike, or driving. For people with brain injuries, procedural memory can be a valuable asset. Even if other memory systems are impacted, procedural memory often remains intact, providing a sense of familiarity and independence. Re-engaging with these skills can be therapeutic, helping the brain reconnect with routine actions.

> **Research Insight:** The basal ganglia and cerebellum are central to procedural memory. Studies have shown that these areas are highly active when people perform repetitive tasks. For example, a study by Doyon found that people who practiced motor skills had increased activation in the cerebellum and basal ganglia, showing their key roles in learned motor activities. [46]

2. Emotional Memory: Emotional **memory** influences how we react based on past experiences. It's why certain places feel calming, or why certain situations make us feel anxious. Emotional memory is stored largely in the amygdala, which connects memories with feelings. Brain injuries can heighten emotional responses, as parts of the brain related to emotion may become more sensitive. Recovery can involve learning techniques like mindfulness and grounding exercises to adjust how we emotionally respond.

> **Research Insight**: Emotional memory is closely linked to the amygdala, especially in how it connects emotions to memories. A study in 1996 found that the amygdala's activity during emotional experiences strengthens memory retention, suggesting it helps "tag" memories with emotional significance, which can be especially pronounced after trauma. [47]

3. Innate Memory: This type of memory manages our most basic, automatic responses, like reflexes and survival instincts. It's why we instinctively react to danger or experience the fight-or-flight response. For some brain injury survivors, the innate memory system can become overly sensitive, leading to increased stress responses to harmless stimuli. Techniques like deep breathing and meditation can help calm this system, retraining the brain to feel safe in daily settings.

> **Research Insight**: The brainstem and amygdala are primary centers for innate memory, coordinating rapid, reflexive responses to perceived threats. Studies on the fight-or-flight response have shown increased amygdala activity when the brain detects danger, even when stimuli are benign, especially in people with heightened anxiety or PTSD. [48]

Each type of non-declarative memory plays a unique role in how we respond to and engage with our world, often acting as a foundation for recovery by maintaining essential skills, reactions, and survival instincts.

Actionable Steps to Strengthen Each Memory Sub-Type

1. Episodic Memory: "Memory Mapping"

Goal: Strengthen personal recall.
How: Choose a memorable event and write down all the details you remember. All the sounds, sights, emotions. Reflect and try to recall more details.
Why: Stimulates the prefrontal cortex and strengthens episodic memory retrieval.

2. Semantic Memory: "Fact Reinforcement"

Goal: Strengthens factual knowledge.
How: Pick a topic, research a fact, and create flashcards. Review them daily.
Why: Repetition and active recall strengthen semantic memory.

3. Prospective Memory: "Reminder System"

Goal: Remember future tasks.
How: List tasks and set alarms or reminders throughout the day. Check off tasks as you complete them.
Why: Engages the prefrontal cortex and hippocampus to remember future actions.

4. Procedural Memory: "Muscle Memory Re-Engagement"

Goal: Re-engage in a learned skill.
How: Practice a motor skill (e.g., typing, cycling) for 10-15 minutes daily, focusing on the steps.
Why: Reinforces neural pathways in the basal ganglia and

cerebellum.

5. Emotional Memory: "Mindfulness Reflection"

Goal: Regulate emotional memory.
How: Reflect on an emotional memory, notice physical sensations, and reframe it positively.
Why: Helps regulate emotions tied to memories by engaging the amygdala.

6. Innate Memory: "Fight-or-Flight Calm Down"

Goal: Calm the stress response.
How: Practice deep breathing (inhale for 4, exhale for 4) and relax your body from head to toe.
Why: Activates the parasympathetic system to calm the amygdala and brainstem.

These exercises are designed to be quick, easy to integrate into daily life, and a holistic support memory improvement and recovery.

Memory Reconsolidation

Memories are like a little story your brain keeps safe for you! Maybe you have a memory of your favorite birthday party, a vacation with your family, or even times when you experienced intense moments of trauma. Your brain is amazing because it keeps all these memories stored away, kind of like dusty books in a library.

We all carry memories. Some are light and joyful, and others might feel heavy and painful. The way we hold onto those memories can impact how we feel every day, but what if you could lighten that burden? **Now, you might think that a memory is a memory, and it stays the same forever, but guess what? They don't!** Memories can change a little bit every time we remember them. That's what scientists call **memory reconsolidation**, a fancy way of saying your brain updates old memories over time, even if you don't know it. Your magnificent brain is constantly working behind the scenes, reshaping and fine-tuning the way those stories are stored.

But here's something even cooler: **You can change a memory on purpose and with intent!** Let's say you think about a time when you felt sad or scared. When you remember it, your brain opens it up, like taking a book off a shelf. Then, you can add new, happy thoughts or feelings to that memory before your brain puts it back. This is called **memory modification**, and it's like being the head librarian of your own memories. **Now this isn't about tricking yourself or into denying that something didn't happen. Absolutely not**! What we are doing here is modifying the memory so that it no longer holds you back in life. Instead of carrying the emotional weight of a bad memory, you're lightening the load. You're freeing up energy and removing the emotional quotient of a traumatic memory.

This may sound like **science fiction** or something off **Star Trek**, but it **works!**

This amazing process is exactly what I use to help people from all over the world within my one-on-one work and group coaching sessions. **I've seen it lead to unimaginable, rapid, and incredible shifts of identity for my patients and with myself.** It's truly a breathtaking experience as a coach to watch someone transform as they let go of the grip that a painful memory once had on them.

What's equally powerful is how this work creates a **ripple effect**. When you change just one memory, belief or perception about yourself, whether it's tied to your identity or your self-worth, it's like **flipping a switch in your brain**. That one change can start to impact everything else in your life, opening new possibilities you may never have thought were possible.

This practice changed my life.

What I have shared with you above is the **mental ju-jitsu** that I used to overcome an extremely traumatic timeframe in my life and ultimately muster up the courage to write this book and share it with you. I have practiced many hours of **memory modification** to help me **leave the past in the past, where it belongs.**

The **ripple effect** occurs when you change one deeply held belief, thought or perception about your identity and sense of self, it **changes your life!**

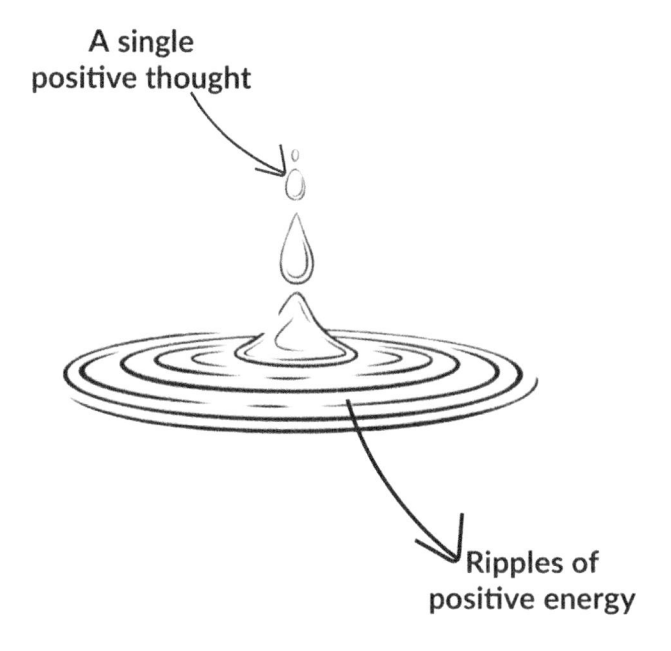

A single positive thought

Ripples of positive energy

The traditional medical system looks at the human mind and body in a linear way. **That A+B must equal C.** If someone has a certain list of symptoms, then it must be that they have a particular type of disease. And if they have a particular form of a disease, we must give them this type of pill.

Can you see how this type of thinking causes more problems than it solves? It's time to shift gears!

Your memory is more powerful and interconnected than you think! Every small step you take to strengthen it helps rebuild not just your brain but your confidence and independence. Over my years of working with brain injury survivors and researching neuroplasticity, I've witnessed how harnessing these memory systems can change lives. I've walked this path myself, and I know recovery is possible with the right tools, understanding, application, and persistence. The brain is always growing, always adapting, and with the right guid-ance, **you can unlock your Inner Warrior within you. Remember you got this!**

Upgrade Your Brain Rescue Journey! VIPs enjoy exclusive early access, massive discounts, and free tools to improve memory. Visit www.dr-bro.com/vipbrainrescue or scan the QR code.

CITATIONS

[1] D'Amato F, Pichiorri F, Tranquillini S, Guglielmelli E, Cincotti F. Guiding breathing at the resonance frequency with haptic sensors potentiates cardiac coherence. Sensors. 2023;23(9):4494. doi: 10.3390/s23094494.

[2] Lally P, Van Jaarsveld CHM, Potts HWW, Wardle J. How are habits formed: Modelling habit formation in the real world. *Eur J Soc Psychol*. 2010;40(6):998-1009. doi:10.1002/ejsp.674

[3] Butler T, Zhou L, Ozsahin I, Wang XH, Garetti J, Zetterberg H, Blennow K, Jamison K, de Leon MJ, Li Y, et al. Glymphatic clearance estimated using diffusion tensor imaging along perivascular spaces is reduced after traumatic brain injury and correlates with plasma neurofilament light, a biomarker of injury severity. Brain Commun. 2023;5(3). doi: 10.1093/braincomms/fcad134.

[4] Neurolaunch. Sleep deprivation vs. drunk: How sleep deprivation can impair cognitive performance like alcohol. Neurolaunch. Available from: https://neurolaunch.com/sleep-deprivation-vs-drunk/

[5] Marta C, Fischer S, Rusu I, et al. Glial cell-derived neurotrophic factor (GDNF) in brain injury. *Neurochem Res*. 2005;30(6):809-16. doi: 10.1007/s11064-005-9020-2.

[6] Lin CY, Lin KP, Hsueh MC, Liao Y. Associations of accelerometer-measured sedentary behavior and physical activity with sleep in older adults. *Clinical Nutrition*. 2023. Available from: https://www.sciencedirect.com/science/article/pii/S0929664623002966

[7] Pennington L, Davie G, Macniven D, et al. Aerobic exercise in mild traumatic brain injury: A systematic review and case study. *Front Hum Neurosci*. 2023;17:10771390. Available from: https://www.frontiersin.org/articles/10.3389/fnhum.2023.1307507/full.

[8] Erickson KI, Voss MW, Prakash R, et al. Exercise training increases size of hippocampus and improves memory. Proc Natl Acad Sci U S A. 2011 May 3;108(18):3017-22. doi: 10.1073/pnas.1015895108.: https://www.pnas.org/doi/full/10.1073/pnas.1015895108

[9] Zhang Y, Cullum CM, Tomoto T, et al. Exercise boosts blood flow to the brain, study finds. UT Southwestern Newsroom. 2023. Available from: https://www.utsouthwestern.edu/newsroom/articles/year-2023/exercise-brain-blood-flow.html

[10] Centers for Disease Control and Prevention. Exposure to glyphosate in the United States: Data from the 2013–2014 National Health and Nutrition Examination Survey. *Environment International*. 2022 Nov 3. Available from: https://www.cdc.gov/biomonitoring/glyphosate.html

[11] Piano, D. A., & Schulz, R. (2012). The influence of mental rehearsal on motor learning: A comparison of physical practice and mental practice. *BMC Neuroscience*, 13, 32. https://doi.org/10.1186/1471-2202-13-32.

[12] Mori K, Inatomi S, Ouchi K, et al. The effect of Hericium erinaceus (Yamabushitake) on cognitive function in mice. *J Ethnopharmacol.* 2009;121(1):20-27.

[13] National Institutes of Health (NIH), Office of Dietary Supplements. Omega-3 Fatty Acids Fact Sheet for Consumers [Internet]. Available from: https://ods.od.nih.gov/pdf/factsheets/Omega3FattyAcids-Consumer.pdf

[14] Anand P, Kunnumakkara AB, Newman RA, Aggarwal BB. Bioavailability of curcumin: Problems and promises. *Mol Pharm.* 2007;4(6):807-818. doi:10.1021/mp700113r.

[15] Centers for Disease Control and Prevention. National Health and Nutrition Examination Survey: Dietary Guidelines [Internet]. Atlanta (GA): CDC; [cited 2024 Nov 25]. Available from: https://www.cdc.gov/nchs/nhanes.htm

[16] Maharaj V, Chowdhury F, Pereira D. Ginkgo biloba and its potential for cognitive enhancement: a review of the clinical evidence. Curr Drug Targets. 2013;14(13):1667-79.

[17] Parletta N, Milte CM, Meyer B, et al. The role of B vitamins in the prevention of dementia: A review of evidence. Oxford Academic; 2020. Available from: https://academic.oup.com/

[18] Harvard Health Publishing. The gut-brain connection [Internet]. Boston (MA): Harvard Medical School; 2023 [cited 2024 Nov 27]. Available from: https://www.health.harvard.edu/diseases-and-conditions/the-gut-brain-connection

[19] Woollett K, Maguire EA. Acquiring "the Knowledge" of London's Layout Drives Structural Brain Changes. *Curr Biol.* 2011 Dec 6;21(23). doi: 10.1016/j.cub.2011.11.018.

[20] Emmons RA, McCullough ME. The impact of gratitude journaling on memory formation and recall. Front Psychol. 2017;8:1349.

[21] Zhou X, Wu M, Liu W, et al. Neural basis of the relationship between ventromedial prefrontal cortex and emotional regulation. Front Psychol. 2015;6:1491. Available from: https://www.frontiersin.org/journals/psychology/articles/10.3389/fpsyg.2015.01491/full

[22] Katsumi Y, Wong B, Cavallari M, Fong TG, Alsop DC, Andreano JM, Carvalho N, Brickhouse M, Jones R, Liberman TA, et al. Structural integrity of the anterior midcingulate cortex contributes to resilience to delirium in SuperAging. *Brain Commun.* 2022;4(4):fcac162. doi:10.1093/braincomms/fcac163.

[23] Brown S. *Play: How it Shapes the Brain, Opens the Imagination, and Invigorates the Soul.* New York: Avery; 2009.

[24] Zhang Y, Li Y, Zhao J, et al. Neural mechanisms of voluntary and involuntary control of breathing. J Neurosci. 2016;36(49):12448-12457. Available from: https://www.jneurosci.org/content/36/49/12448

[25] Nielson EL, Kothari K, Johansen J, et al. The effects of intermittent hypoxic training on the cardiovascular system. Chest. 2017;151(5):1137-1148. Available from: https://journal.chestnet.org/article/S0012-3692(16)52386-1/abstract

[26] Mental Health Explorer. The neuroscience of happiness. *Mental Health Explorer.* Available from: https://www.mentalhealthexplorer.org/articles/the-neuroscience-of-happiness

[27] Minecheck. Your brain is processing more data than you would ever imagine. *Minecheck*. Available from: https://www.minecheck.com/posts/your-brain-is-processing-more-data-than-you-would-ever-imagine/

[28] Association for Psychological Science. Your brain sees even when you don't. *Psychological Science*. Available from: https://www.psychologicalscience.org/news/your-brain-sees-even-when-you-dont.html

[29] Harvard University. Study on mindfulness meditation and brain changes. *Harvard Study*. Available from: https://www.sog.unc.edu/sites/default/files/course_materials/HARVARD-STUDY2014-ON-MEDITATION.pdf

[30] Findlay, J. M. Express saccades and visual attention. *Behavioral and Brain Sciences*. Available from: https://www.cambridge.org/core/journals/behavioral-and-brain-sciences/article/abs/express-saccades-and-visual-attention/B38F6BA1820BDD8753880DCD2814AC7D

[31] Johns Hopkins Medicine. Brain response study upends thinking about why practice speeds up motor reaction times [Internet]. 2018 Aug 16 [cited 2024 Nov 29]. Available from: https://www.hopkinsmedicine.org/news/newsroom/news-releases/2018/08/brain-response-study-upends-thinking-about-why-practice-speeds-up-motor-reaction-times

[32] Van Nuland SE, Rogers WA. A current view on dual-task paradigms and their limitations to capture cognitive load. Front Hum Neurosci [Internet]. 2016 [cited 2024 Nov 29]; 10:583. Available from: https://www.frontiersin.org/articles/10.3389/fnhum.2016.00583/full

[33] National Eye Institute. Activity in brain system that controls eye movements highlights importance of spatial thinking. National Eye Institute. 2024 Sep 19. Available from: https://www.nei.nih.gov/research/activities-research/news/2024/09/19/brain-system-eye-movements-importance-spatial-thinking:contentReference{index=0}.

[34] Frontiers in Neurology. A comprehensive review of neural mechanisms underlying auditory processing and its effects on cognitive function. Front Neurol. 2023. Available from: https://www.frontiersin.org/journals/neurology/articles/10.3389/fneur.2023.1122420/full:contentReference{index=0}.

[35] Smith PF, Darlington CL. Vestibular system and memory. *Front Integr Neurosci*. 2014;8:59. Available from: https://www.frontiersin.org/journals/integrative-neuroscience/articles/10.3389/fnint.2014.00059/full

[36] Mark G, Gudith D, Klocke U. The cost of interrupted work: More speed and stress. *Proceedings of the SIGCHI Conference on Human Factors in Computing Systems*. 2008:107–10. DOI:10.1145/1357054.1357072.

[37] PPM Express. Context switching: how it kills productivity and how to reduce it [Internet]. 2024 [cited 2024 Nov 30]. Available from: https://ppm.express/blog/context-switching/

[38] American Psychological Association. Multitasking: Switching costs. Available from: https://www.apa.org/topics/research/multitasking

[39] Assaraf J, Smith M. *The Secret*. Page 48.

[40] Lv S, Wu J, Zhang D, Wu X, Song H, Peng L, et al. Transcutaneous auricular vagus

nerve stimulation for treatment-resistant depression: A randomized, sham-controlled trial. *Front Neurol.* 2022;13:1030927. doi:10.3389/fneur.2022.1030927.

[41] ZenRji. Research. ZenRji. Available from: https://www.zenrji.uk/research

[42] Binnewijzend MA, Kuijer JPA, Eppink N, et al. Cerebral blood flow and cognitive functioning in a community-based, multi-ethnic cohort: The SABRE study. *Front Neurol.* 2020;11:984. doi:10.3389/fnins.2020.00984.

[43] Kapur S, Craik FI, Jones C, Brown GM, Houle S, Tulving E. Functional role of the prefrontal cortex in retrieval of memories: a PET study. Neuroreport. 1995;6(14):1880-4.

[44] Binder JR, Desai RH, Graves WW, Conant LL. Where is the semantic system? A critical review and meta-analysis of 120 functional neuroimaging studies. Cereb Cortex. 2009;19(12):2767-96.

[45] McDaniel MA, Einstein GO. Strategic and automatic processes in prospective memory retrieval: A multiprocess framework. Appl Cogn Psychol. 2000;14(7)

[46] Doyon J, et al. Contributions of the basal ganglia and functionally related brain structures to motor learning. Behav Brain Res. 2009;199(1):61-75.

[47] Cahill L, et al. Amygdala activity at encoding correlated with long-term, free recall of emotional information. Proc Natl Acad Sci U S A. 1996;93(15):8016-21.

[48] LeDoux JE. Emotion circuits in the brain. Annu Rev Neurosci. 2000;23(1):155-84.

ABOUT THE AUTHOR

Dr. Brody Miller, PhD, is one of the leading brain rehabilitation experts in the world and the founder of a global 226,000-strong healing community that is still growing.

Dr. Brody's own story is one of significant struggles with brain health. A few years after a severe traumatic brain injury, neurosurgeons removed a bloody cavernous malformation in Brody's brain that was causing him to have grand mal seizures. At this time, Brody was deeply tormented by the wounds from his past, and in his own words, "he was once a walking disaster." This painful journey led him to discover neuroplasticity and the brain's incredible ability to heal itself.

At the heart of Dr. Brody's work is the *R.E.B.O.U.N.D Method™*, a holistic, natural approach to brain healing that empowers patients to rewire their brains without risky surgeries or harmful medications.

When Brody's not crafting new mind gym exercises or helping others on their brain health healing journey, he can be found exercising, meditating in nature, reading, and traveling the world! Dr Brody absolutely loves animals, especially dogs. Brody lives in a majestic mountain town near Denver, USA, with his loving wife Rocio, and big black-brown rescue dog, Heart.

Dr. Brody Miller's overall mission is simple yet profound: to help empower brain recovery warriors to rewrite their stories, push past their limits, and ultimately "become their own doctor".

Take the next step in your recovery:

- Follow Dr. Brody on Instagram and other social media channels: @DrBrodyMiller
- Watch his educational videos on YouTube: https://www.youtube.com/@drbrodymiller
- Explore free resources and learn more: (Insert Authority Funnel Link)

Also, absolutely make sure to sign up to my **VIP email list** to get **exclusive early access** and **huge discounts** on upcoming offers by going to **www.dr-bro.com/vipbrainrescue or** scanning the QR code below.

Printed in Great Britain
by Amazon